Mom's Losing Her Memory
I'm Losing My Mind!

Taking Care of Mom and Dad
with Memory Decline

Kathy Jean Stewart RN, BSN

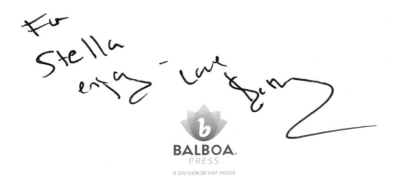

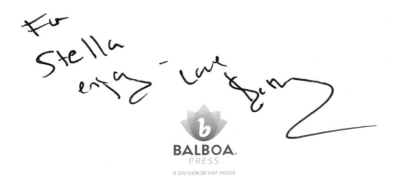
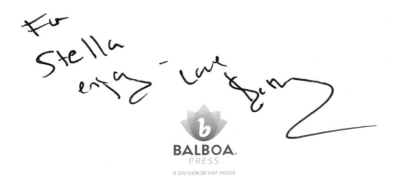

BALBOA
PRESS

A DIVISION OF HAY HOUSE

Balboa Press books may be ordered through booksellers or by contacting:

Balboa Press
A Division of Hay House
1663 Liberty Drive
Bloomington, IN 47403
www.balboapress.com
1-(877) 407-4847

Because of the dynamic nature of the Internet, any web addresses or links contained in this book may have changed since publication and may no longer be valid. The views expressed in this work are solely those of the author and do not necessarily reflect the views of the publisher, and the publisher hereby disclaims any responsibility for them.

The author of this book does not dispense medical advice or prescribe the use of any technique as a form of treatment for physical, emotional, or medical problems without the advice of a physician, either directly or indirectly. The intent of the author is only to offer information of a general nature to help you in your quest for emotional and spiritual well-being. In the event you use any of the information in this book for yourself, which is your constitutional right, the author and the publisher assume no responsibility for your actions.

Editorial assistance: Elly Trepman, M.D. (manuscriptsurgeon.com)

Cover: Gayle Kagen

Printed in the United States of America

ISBN: 978-1-4525-6933-8 (sc)
ISBN: 978-1-4525-6935-2 (hc)
ISBN: 978-1-4525-6934-5 (e)

Library of Congress Control Number: 2013903395

Balboa Press rev. date: 03/19/2013

Mom's Losing Her Memory, I'm Losing My Mind! is written by a nurse who shares her experiences in an assisted living environment, providing invaluable insight and guidance in caring for Mom and Dad who are aging with dementia.

To my father,

Marshall James Schwarzbach,

who gave me the strength and perseverance

to succeed in my life purpose:

assisting others with situations of declining health.

TABLE OF CONTENTS

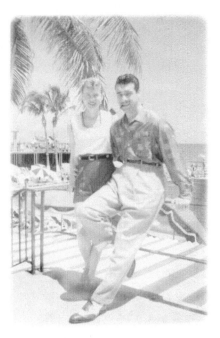

Preface

My Path to Caring for the Elderly

The "seed" for my interest in caring for the elderly was first planted years ago when I was in middle school. During that time, three of my grandparents were experiencing a significant decline in their health.

My maternal grandfather had been a World War I veteran, engaged in many major ground battles during his tour in the war. Unfortunately, he was exposed to mustard gas during the war, and doctors believed that this contributed to his fast mental decline with dementia. He had rapid loss of cognitive abilities, and he experienced hallucinations and delusions. At times he became very violent, as if he still was fighting in the war. I was curious and disturbed by his condition, eager to learn how and why this was happening to my grandfather. I wanted to know how we might best handle his symptoms, but there was very little information or direction for care available.

My grandfather endured a long stay in the hospital for veterans, where he was constantly sedated and secured to his bed with wrist and body restraints. This hospital reeked of unpleasant odors and was very stark and unappealing. I remember dreading the visits to my grandfather at the hospital because it seemed like such a horrible place. Before his decline, my grandfather weighed 180 pounds, but near the end of his life, he weighed only ninety pounds. My mother and grandmother visited him daily, bringing him milk shakes with the hope that he would gain weight. Although his treatment was standard practice, I knew that there must be a better way to care for his illness.

Soon after my grandfather passed away, my grandmother began to have memory loss. I know that the emotional and physical stress of dealing with my grandfather's illness contributed to my grandmother's decline. My mother chose to care for her in our home, but it was not easy. Although my grandmother was more lucid and independent than my grandfather had been, there were countless occasions when she left the water running, causing a flood in the bathroom. Sometimes she forgot to turn off the stove-top gas, which was dangerous for the entire family. We loved her deeply, but the constant care and attention that my grandmother required was a big stress to my mother. Yet it was important for her to help my grandmother avoid a facility that had been so frightening for my grandfather.

At this time, my father's mother was also declining. She had a very sharp memory, but she experienced physical decline because of heart disease and general weakness. She needed care with every aspect of dressing, bathing, and getting around. My parents chose to place her in an assisted living community with experts on site to provide care for her mounting physical needs. The assisted living environment was safe and homelike, without nasty odors. I remember looking forward to visiting her at the assisted living home for ice-cream socials or musical events, and eventually she died there after many years of great care.

After this intimate exposure to different types of care for the elderly, it became my life purpose to help the elderly in a compassionate and respectful way. Sure enough, I became a registered nurse. Entering the nursing profession allowed me to pursue a meaningful career in which I could give to the elderly in a purposeful way. I discovered that I deeply enjoyed interacting with the senior population, tackling the challenges of managing their complex health-care needs.

After many years of working as a nurse in various health-care settings, I developed the skills of a persistent detective, enabling me to identify symptoms and manage them effectively. As a director of a well-respected assisted living community, I am very proud to provide effective care for elderly residents, especially those with dementia. It has been gratifying that family members have often commented on the improved quality of their parent's physical and mental well-being.

This book shares the knowledge that I have gleaned over the years, working with the elderly and their families. My hope is that the stories and suggestions in this book will benefit the many grown children and spouses who are suddenly confronted with the overwhelming challenge of caring for an elderly family member. There still may be some happy times, even for those with dementia or memory loss. This book is intended to help people understand and develop skills in all aspects of elderly care.

Introduction

From the time we were young, many of us envisioned a future that included getting married and having children. We may have pictured our parents living nearby and serving as affectionate grandparents, eager to assist us with the next generation. Holidays would be spent with our parents and children happily having meals around a dining room table filled with food, laughter, love, and great conversation. After the delightfully lavish holiday meals, the extended family would gather around board games, and our healthy, clearheaded parents would entertain their grandkids with funny stories about our childhood.

Unfortunately, this is not a reality experienced by most people. When the time comes for us to start our own families, we may find ourselves living far from our parents. Visits to the grandparents may be infrequent because of the pressures of work, school schedules, and the cost of travel. Telephone conversations are short and redundant: "How are you?" "How is work?" "How is school?" "What are you studying?" This is far from the picture-perfect world we had imagined as children, back in the "good old days."

Today, a more typical scene might look like this: Grandma and

Grandpa are visiting for a special holiday meal. After some yelling up the stairs, or calling our children's cell phones to get them to the table, the meal begins with conversation in "sound bites." Family members are distracted by thoughts of the next place they need to be or are mentally consumed by their challenging days. Suddenly, Grandma begins to call family members by the wrong names, and she does not remember her daughter-in-law. That gets everyone's attention!

After the daughter-in-law is identified, Grandma is in disbelief that her son has been married for twenty-five years, because she still sees him as twenty-five years old. The final straw is an emotional outburst from Grandpa, or maybe the sudden realization that Grandma needs a change of clothing because she soiled her pants.

The gradual decline of the aging grandparents continues. The phone calls are no longer conversations about family concerns or world matters. They are crisis-prevention calls with repeated questions, such as: "Have you eaten today?" or "Did you take your pills?" Your parents call you "honey" more than your given name, and you wonder if they actually recognize you.

On the good days, conversations focus on general small talk. Nothing specific or personal is mentioned, because there is no short-term memory to carry the conversation. Mom and Dad cannot remember that they just called you, so you receive calls that are more and more frequent. Nights have no boundaries, and the calls happen at all hours of the night because Mom and Dad cannot sleep.

Finally, you decide to visit Mom and Dad's home, and you determine that the family must intervene. You find no food in the refrigerator. The shower, washer, and dryer are not being used. Your parents once maintained a high standard of personal hygiene, and now this is lost. Dad is wearing clothing with multiple food stains, and he has body odor. Mom has bruises on her knees, forearms, and forehead from a fall, but when questioned, she does not remember what happened. They used to love to cook, and their refrigerator had always been filled with gourmet leftovers; now you discover that even canned or frozen foods are not being used. Your parents are thinner because they are losing weight. They need help … from you!

Mom and Dad always took care of you. How is it possible that you must take care of them? Day care was easy for the kids, but it is very different to take charge of Mom and Dad's physical health and well-being. Where do you start? How do you do this?

My goal is to share with you the unforeseen circumstance of caring for parents as they age and develop memory loss and dementia. We will cover:

» the challenges of maintaining or building a relationship with your parents as they become more confused and in need;

» how to tackle the issues of maintaining your life and sanity as you grasp the reality of caring for your parents (and your children at the same time);

» practical ways to carry on with your life and fulfill your commitment to your parents;

» elderly decline and care needs from a nursing perspective, primarily in the assisted living environment;

» examples of real-life situations, with names changed to protect the privacy of the individuals;

» nutritional support for maintaining optimum health throughout the aging process;

» the fact that you are not alone and that support and resources are available.

CHAPTER 1

Prelude to Dementia

Alice, who is eighty-three years old, sits in an elderly care community with her eyes closed, listening to a voice telling her to open her mouth and take another bite. Alice keeps her mouth closed in protest. She does not want to ingest another bit of food. Alice has lost fifteen pounds during advanced stages of Alzheimer's dementia, a disease she has been battling for eight years. She also has lost her ability to walk independently, and she is weak and unsteady. She is confined to a wheelchair for safety.

The persistent voice of her daughter, Gretchen, once again demands that she should open her mouth and take a bite of dinner. Gretchen, now in her fifties, is searching for distant memories of when she was young and this role was reversed. She tries to remember the tricks her mother used to get her to open her mouth.

Gretchen recalls a time when she herself was ill and very dehydrated. Her mother would hold a spoonful of clear soup and beg Gretchen to open her mouth, promising her a new outfit after she got better. "Mom," Gretchen explains, "if you eat and get stronger, we can go shopping!" Alice's mouth remains closed.

Gretchen is losing patience. "Open your eyes!" she demands. Gretchen looks into her mother's blue eyes, hoping to find a spark of attentiveness. Instead, she gazes into what seem to be the eyes of a distant stranger who has no interest in Gretchen or what she is saying.

Gretchen has had a long day at work and is tired. She wonders what food she has at home to make dinner for herself and her husband, who by now is probably waiting for her at home. She turns to Alice, who is very thin and does not resemble the able-bodied mother who raised her. She wants her mother to eat, regain strength, and return to a time when she could remember Gretchen's identity.

Alzheimer's disease has taken Alice from Gretchen, but Gretchen wants her mom back. Occasionally, Alice may be more bright-eyed and experience moments of clear memory, lucid thoughts, and conversation. However, these times pass, and Alice returns to a state of not knowing her daughter Gretchen at all. Alice then repeatedly asks questions about where her long-deceased parents are located, and she reflects on their recent visit. Gretchen does not know how to handle these statements about parents who died many years ago and thoughts that are not reality.

Gretchen's eyes fill with tears as she struggles with this overwhelming and frustrating responsibility. How does this happen? Why is it happening to Alice? What is the best way to care for her? Who has the answers? Gretchen knows she is not the first person to encounter this situation, but it is the first time for her, and she is lost.

Little guidance is provided for many typical journeys and challenges in life. Surprises are around every corner along life's most important paths. Why are we surprised? Why is there not more guidance before big events in life, such as childbirth? I remember thinking during my first experience giving birth, and all the new experiences that followed, that there is too much unshared information. Much of what happens to us throughout the generations is not discussed.

Despite the difficulties of raising children, many people have the passionate opinion that their experience of raising children was their most significant accomplishment. The small print should read, "With the child-rearing experience, you may encounter sleepless nights, emotional upset, financial stress, and other disturbances." Although literature is available for advice, most sources are inexact and contain theories and opinions that may not apply to the situation. This may cause anxiety about not doing it correctly. For example, timeouts never worked with my children. I tried this many ways and read how it should work if done correctly. My children just got up any time they pleased. The magnitude of the responsibility, experience, formal hands-on instruction, and guidance were lacking in the raising and guiding of children. The unfortunate first-child syndrome should be labeled experimental-child syndrome, defined as *when* the parents learn. This critical information about child care and rearing responsibility is transmitted through self-study at home with books, the Internet, and parenting magazines.

The surprises and challenges in life do not end with child rearing. Another hidden reality that goes unspoken is the secret of what actually may happen when we finally get our children to a stage when there is not as much physical and directional work anymore. The kids are more independent, and family activities evolve, so the child and adult become more connected through conversations and negotiations. We dream this day will come, but it arrives with the surprise of yet another unspoken reality for which we may not be prepared.

We become blindsided by the care of Mom and Dad and have no preparation for this monster of new responsibility. We find ourselves fumbling through issues with little guidance. A new, learn-as-you-go experience now faces us when we must care for aging parents.

More Responsibility

A typical day for the working family with young children is jam-packed. After a full day of work from 9:00 a.m. to 5:00 p.m., the parents tackle the children's after-school activities that may include soccer games, basketball practice, and gymnastics meets. After these activities, we may require a quick stop at the grocery store before preparing dinner. That is the life of the many baby boomers who juggle kids and work. Just when you think there is no room for any more responsibilities, you are suddenly faced with the task of taking care of your parents.

How do you fit another responsibility into your day? If there was a choice, the time would be spent planning and taking a vacation. However, why bother contemplating a vacation when you now have the additional worry of coordinating the care of your parents when you are out of town?

In the past, people lived shorter lives. However, nutrition and health care have advanced over the years, enabling people to live longer. Previously, the elderly died from heart failure, cancers, and infections that were not treated so progressively. In the new age of more advanced health care, an abundance of healthier foods, and improved diagnostic tests, our bodies may live longer than before.

With so many physical needs addressed by today's health care, why is it that Alzheimer's dementia and memory disorders are more prevalent? As our bodies persevere longer with modern health care, our minds seem to deteriorate. Dementia is the loss of brain function that progresses from mild memory loss ("senior moments") to more severe loss of memory, thought processes, language, judgment, and normal behavior.

In many people, the health of the mind does not keep up with that of the body. The brain may continue to deteriorate faster than the other parts of the body, but the patient receives medication and assistive devices that do not keep the mind working. We often successfully mend the body, but how can we mend the mind? This problem is clearly identified, but it has no solution.

Mom is physically healthy, but as she ages, her brain is dying. As her mind function is lost, she cannot care for herself, and she is unable to learn new skills that are necessary in a constantly changing world. Rarely do you see the elderly in the self-scan checkout line in a grocery store, using a bank machine, speaking on a cell phone, or paying bills online. It is a good day when you do not need to help Mom with the television controls. As technology speeds ahead, the elderly do not keep up, and they cannot manage previously familiar tasks.

Therefore, the adult children must step up and do something to help. In past generations, aging parents would move into their homes. With fewer divorces in the past, and in most cases, mothers at home raising families, the environment was more conducive to taking in the aging parent. Now, stay-at-home moms are rarely at home. They are in the car, driving a constant child shuttle, and in most cases, nobody is at home full-time. Moms are working to attempt to collectively meet the mounting financial needs of raising a family in today's costly and complex society.

For the baby boomer generation, taking in a parent is a much different struggle than in the past, because nobody is at home to watch the parent. Parents might need help, and out of guilt or perhaps a sense of inherited commitment, many adult children try to take their parents into their own homes for assistance and needed care. This challenge most often proves to be a nightmare. Safety becomes an issue; leaving Dad alone in the home becomes the safety equivalent of leaving a toddler at home alone. Now you are the one directing your parent, but arguments and frustrations ensue. Dad may not remember much, but he does remember that he is your parent, and in his mind, you should obey him.

I often meet with adult children or aged spouses who tour the assisted living community where I work. Many times, the spouses say they are looking for something down the road for their partner. As a nurse, I know this often means "until the next crisis." The person may be holding on to the present situation until the next catastrophic event exceeds what they can handle at home. He or she might be functioning in a gray zone of hanging on and getting through the daily tasks of existence at a very basic level of safety and survival. This situation could change suddenly with a fall or health-care event that makes it impossible for this living situation to continue. This may be the catalyst for making a change and finding an alternative care environment for his or her spouse. However, it is best to plan and prepare for this change before a crisis or emergency.

911 or Bust

Several weeks after Judy toured our community, I received a frantic phone call from her. From the panic in her voice, I could tell that her family was in crisis. At the time of the tour, she was casually evaluating the assisted living community as an option for her mother, Ethel. Even if she determined that assisted living would be the best living situation, she felt it might be months before Ethel would need this transition of care.

Ethel was living in Southern California with Judy's brother, Todd, and his family. Todd was doing everything possible to care for their mom at home and thought this was the "right thing" to do. Ethel did not remember what was being done for her from day to day, but she did remember how to call 911. She began to call this number repeatedly to report that she was being "abused."

Todd and his young family, who were caring for Ethel, were not abusing her at all, but her poor memory led to delusions that seemed very real to her.

Protective services came to investigate. This was the breaking point for Judy's brother. Ethel was being sent from California to live with Judy, who lived in the Seattle area, as soon as possible. However, if Mom's delusions and dialing 911 continued, Judy also would have protective services at her door.

This situation is very common to many families who are adamant about trying to care for their mom or dad at home. Judy needed to recognize that she could not care for Mom by herself at home and that she needed either extra support at home or a different setting, such as an assisted living community.

Devotion until Death

I first met Claire when I cared for her mother years ago in the assisted living community. During that time, Claire was energetic and full of life. She and her husband, Gordon, used to visit her mother several times each week. Claire loved to join her mother for walks, go out for lunch, or visit late in the evening to join in a game of bingo.

Later, Claire returned to the community because she was caring for her husband, ten years her senior. At first, I did not recognize her because she appeared to have aged considerably. She was much thinner than before and appeared exhausted. Her spark of life and high energy, qualities that I had admired, were missing in the new Claire. She sat in my office, voicing her dedication to her husband and their marriage. However, she realized that caring for Gordon at home was wearing her down, and her health was suffering. She wanted to know my opinion about when she should bring her husband to the assisted living setting. Without hesitation, I said, "Now."

This is a common situation because the spouse caregiver may

feel obligated by a marriage vow voiced years ago, and he or she may have a moral bond to the marriage commitment. Some feel the marriage vow is made blindly because of the endless limits of the future unknowns. The spouse caregiver feels she should take care of her declining husband in poor health, even if it now leads to the demise of her own health. "In sickness and in health," as stated in the marriage vows, surely does not mean "to continue with care in the home when that causes a decline in the caregiver's own health."

When saying "I do" and "until death do us part," it generally means "living together forever through life's trials and tribulations." When most couples say the words "I do" under oath, they may envision issues that include broken bones, heart disease, failing eyesight, shared child rearing, and financial challenges. They may envision these joint life challenges to continue through retirement. They may not consider the issues involved in caring for a spouse with dementia or memory loss, including dressing, bathing, and incontinence. Members of the older generations typically feel that they should be living together with their spouse, and they may be reluctant to leave their spouse at a care community. If the marriage contract was revised today, it might be more realistic to say:

"… As you age and become incontinent of bowel and bladder, and your mind deteriorates to the point where you do not remember your spouse or the fact that you are married, you will continue to care for each other. As you age and continue to physically and mentally deteriorate, you will stand by each other in extreme emotional and physical duress and provide for each other's daily care needs. As the care needs spiral down with mental and health inabilities multiplying, you will continue to stay by the side of this declining partner through this hardship until one of you dies first." With a more "true to life" statement, I wonder how many couples would think twice before making this marriage vow.

Claire was exhausted, neglecting her own health and well-being out of commitment to caring for her declining husband. She went from caring for her aging mother to caring for her husband. Claire stopped her daily walks that she had previously enjoyed, for fear that something might happen to Gordon when she left him alone, even for a short time. Claire eventually lost contact with her friends because she could not relax when she went out with them, worrying about what Gordon was doing at home alone.

Claire's declining health, as a consequence of caring for her husband, was confirmed when I questioned her. She had obviously lost weight, had high blood pressure, suffered from back pain from lifting, was taking anti-anxiety medication because of stress, and was on antidepressants because she was experiencing extreme sadness. In contrast, Gordon was in great shape because Claire was doing a fantastic job caring for him. She cried out for assistance with her question, "When is a good time to seek assisted living for Gordon?" For this life situation, she had neither instructions nor orientation. Help was past due, and guidance was needed desperately.

There are very few resources with information about how to care for each stage of adult aging and dementia. It is only in these crisis situations when people become aware of the systems and supports available. At these times, people may turn to organizations and specialists for educational support, such as the Alzheimer's Association, local senior services organizations, or hospital-based social workers. When these services are not effective, we find ourselves in the emergency room with Mom or Dad for a health crisis we cannot manage at home.

Our society is very good at putting systems in place for the crisis event. However, we need new systems to best take care of our aging parent in a *preventive* manner. Health issues can be addressed with appropriate health care to avoid the crisis 911 call and the emergency room visit. Unfortunately, at present, crisis management may be the only available health-care support for the aging parent.

This lack of awareness and direction leaves most people feeling blindsided as they make their way through uncharted territory. There is little direction on how to prevent the many crisis situations that eventually evolve, such as when Dad has delusions and accuses you of stealing his assets, or when you find he has wandered out in the middle of the night and is lost. Most of us are left to fight through our own experiences to figure out how to best provide care for Mom and Dad's safety.

It is a reality check to consider that this person you are caring for is your mother, the one who guided you on your first steps, potty trained you, and held back dessert if you did not eat your dinner. You now find yourself holding back Mom's dessert because that is all she wants to eat, despite her declining state of nutrition. The guidance situations are similar, but now your roles are reversed.

Those who care for a spouse with dementia may find themselves relishing memories of a life from the past when they raised the kids, bought their first home, and enjoyed adventures and vacations. Sadly, the spouse with dementia does not remember this life or these experiences. At times, he or she may not even recognize the spouse, who becomes very lonely. There may be comfort in photograph albums, but this remains the only viable documentation that the remembered past events actually occurred.

This was the husband who stood by your side, once a partner in decisions, for whom you now make all the decisions. This man, for whom you now provide elder care, needs constant physical care, challenges your patience with his memory loss, and pushes you daily to the edge of sanity. Many times, you just wish for one full night of sleep without getting up and wondering where he went, or whether you need to toilet him again.

It is the caregiver who fights through the constant random situations, not knowing what will be next. The caregiver bears the most wear and tear and feels the most impact of stress. Then the desperate caregiver enters our assisted living community and asks, "When should Mom, Dad, or my spouse enter the assisted living environment?" When this happens, my usual response is, "Now."

What Is Dementia?

Dementia is a term that includes many diseases that affect the function and thought processes of the brain. It is more than just about "forgetting" or any other normal part of aging. It affects all of the following brain functions:

- » thought process
- » ability to process language
- » speech
- » behavior
- » perceptions and emotions

Types of Dementia

The most common type of dementia is Alzheimer's disease:

- » Nerves in the brain are damaged.
- » There is no cure.
- » Treatment includes drugs that may treat symptoms of behaviors and emotions or improve nerve function.

Other types of dementia include:

- » **Lewy Body Dementia:** This dementia is caused by abnormal protein structures in the brain. People with this dementia typically have problems with body movements and hallucinations.

» **Vascular Dementia:** This is caused by strokes or blood clots that prevent blood flow to cells in the brain.

Symptoms most common to many of the dementias:

» The brain shrinks, with loss of function.

» Initially, recent memories are lost; eventually, long-term memories fade.

» Thought processes are difficult, including reasoning and making sense of something.

» Communication is difficult. Initially, it may be difficult to find the right word; later, there is difficulty communicating an entire thought.

» Emotions are difficult to control and exaggerated in some situations.

» Loss of movement control can cause clumsy and unsteady walking, with occasional falls.

» Thought processes are abnormal and may include delusions.

» Paranoid thoughts occur.

The Good, the Bad, the Ugly

The Good:

» Drugs are available to improve brain activity and treat symptoms of depression, primarily in the early stages.

» A good family history of activities for staying alert, such as doing brain activities and interacting with the environment, may help prevent the loss of brain function.

» Eating healthy foods, taking nutritional supplements, doing regular exercise, and monitoring health situations, such as high blood pressure, may help prevent dementia.

» Some forms of dementia, caused by physiological abnormalities or chemical imbalances, such as abnormal levels of blood sugar, vitamin B12, sodium, and calcium, may be reversible.

The Bad and the Ugly:

» It is not normal.

» It takes away independence.

» It can rob people of their dignity.

» Most dementias are nonreversible.

» Relationships are affected and sometimes ruined.

Where Do We Start?

After reading so many wonderful books about spirituality and various religions, I have my own theories of why we are here and how life takes certain turns. Many people believe that the purpose of life is to learn, grow, and impact others and ourselves in a positive way. So where do dementia and old age fit in with this purpose? How does the decaying of our minds and bodies fit into our quest for a meaningful life?

There is no answer that makes sense for everyone. No science or data can answer the nonmaterial questions about our reality. I can share with you my conclusions from my experiences and daily interactions in elderly care. My belief is that we are here in the present world to improve our core self. During our personal growth in adulthood, we age and may decline, our bodies wilting over time. We develop wrinkles and failing body parts until we are not recognized as the same person from our past. Many people become weak and less vibrant as they age, until they die. However, we are conscious beings, and our recipe for living vibrantly includes the will to live and engage in a purposeful life.

Nevertheless, the path of nurturing, to bloom fully, only to wilt in older age, is a common life course. As human beings, we break away from the simple perspective of physical decline, and we become more conscious and thoughtful. Using our cognitive abilities, we sustain our lives with thoughtful connections. These connections include family support and adult children who can care for us as we age. This reciprocal nurturing pattern from the adult children enables us to age safely as our health declines. Furthermore, these thoughtful connections can evolve, and we learn to enjoy other aspects of our surroundings.

The challenge of supporting the aging mind of people who have dementia is complicated by the physical decline of aging. In contrast with physical decline, which can be seen, the thoughts and actions in a person with a declining mind may take an invisible and unpredictable course, with solutions harder to find.

Our day-to-day thoughts and reactions are based on what we actively and collectively remember from the past and present. We are likely to recall high-impact events that caused extreme physical or emotional feelings, because these memories were so important in our lives. In contrast, we may not remember the less significant experiences that, nonetheless, contributed to our personal identity. With dementia, memories about significant key events become distorted versions of previous happenings. This distorted memory intertwines some aspects of the remembered past with the present reality, creating a version of events that never actually happened.

With long-term memory still intact, Mom may recall bits of reality from long ago. She may remember, as if it were yesterday, the day Dad proposed or intimate details of your birth. She may remember random newsworthy events from the past that were very important to her. During trivia games in the assisted living setting, I find it fascinating how elderly residents with dementia may remember endless random details from the distant past, such as lyrics to a song or dates of a president's death, but may not recall what they ate for lunch that day.

Mom with dementia may develop an alternate, distorted memory that changes the way she feels. She may have a new favorite child, because the past memories about one child are now twisted and are remembered differently. I recall recently speaking to Jasmine, a daughter of a resident, who was thrilled that her father with dementia now remembers her as the perfect daughter. This was a great experience for her, because in the years before the dementia, Jasmine described her father as being judgmental, and she was viewed as the child who could never do anything right.

In another twist of memory with dementia, Dad, who always trusted you with financial advice, remembers events differently, and this triggers him not to trust you. There is no logical way to predict how the mind with dementia works and how Dad currently remembers details from the past.

Carla called me in tears one day from her home because she was experiencing a visit from the local police. Her father, Russell, had called the police and accused Carla and her husband of stealing from him. Carla and her husband had been caring for Russell for many months, but he seemed to be more confused and forgetful.

Russell seemed composed to the police because he could recite specific details to the officer of how his money was taken from him without his permission. Although the descriptions of stealing were false, Russell believed them to be true. Russell had grown up during the Great Depression, and this may have contributed to his paranoid and distorted version of memory.

Just as past experiences affect Dad's memory as he ages,

his current experiences sculpt perceptions of daily encounters that affect his present mood. Isolation and lack of stimulation can cause depression and withdrawal. Dad's withdrawal from present interactions promote memory decline and may accelerate dementia. Conversely, if Dad is active with interactions he enjoys, he may be more attentive and alert. As the adult child caring for Dad with dementia, you may provide many experiences for him, with the hope of promoting a happy memory and better mental health.

Chapter 2

Embracing the Unknown—Dementia

The Best Approach to Dementia:
Preventing the "Wilting of the Mind"

My intention for elderly care is to create a stimulating and positive experience for people with dementia, so they may embrace their perception of the world in a happy and healthy way. This recipe for positive influence includes addressing all aspects of Mom's experience in a manner she will embrace. Although I discuss approaches to improve memory, a positive, stimulating approach also may optimize physical function in the elderly. Consistent mind stimulation for the person with dementia will encourage her to use her remaining memory function and may reduce further decline.

Stimulating Mom's memory for improved health is analogous to providing water to sustain the rose wilting with age.

Dad with dementia most likely will not remember many

positive experiences in which he is engaged. However, there may be a benefit of participating in activities to exercise and stimulate the mind and create happiness, even in very advanced stages of memory decline. He may not show any indication of how he enjoys a situation until it is removed, and, as a result, he has a deterioration of behavior. When Dad is removed from a compatible care situation that he enjoyed and then placed in a care situation that he finds less appealing, he will show his displeasure. If he is unable to communicate verbally because of advanced dementia, he may show his disapproval by becoming more anxious, depressed, combative, or withdrawn.

The care environment may change when the patient must move to the hospital, a different nursing home, or a new assisted care situation. Dad may miss his routine or the staff person who loved and cared for him in knowing ways. Dad's fragile health in his elderly state can quickly worsen from depression that develops because of change in care or unhappiness with a new environment. When depressed, he may eat less and withdraw more, and as a result, his health may spiral downward. This additional decline in Dad's health may be the final event that tips his frail state to an end-of-life decline.

Elderly people who experience depression, triggered by a change in environment, may die just months after the change. Ernie was living at home with his wife until he became ill with pneumonia and confusion. After hospitalization, he had a short stay in a nursing home before being transferred to a group home. Ernie did not adjust to these unwanted environmental changes. He missed his house, his wife, and customary foods, and he disliked the new soft diet. Ernie withdrew and did not communicate with his family on visits. Eventually, he was admitted to hospice because of weight loss and decline in health, and he died a few weeks later.

Other changes may be a clear benefit to Dad because he

may find a more compatible environment that makes him happy. Bob was bored and lonely at home, watching television most of the day. He was not motivated to exercise or eat well. Then his daughter brought him to the assisted living community, where he made friends and became more social. He showed up for all meals and regained his weight and good health. The more stimulating and compatible environment provided Bob with the opportunity to thrive, just like the wilting rose that is finally given water.

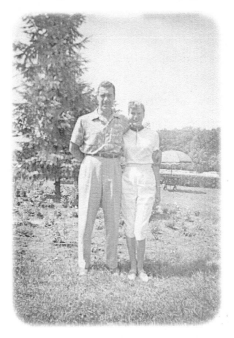

When Reality Hits

Signs that suggest that Dad may have memory loss or dementia include:

» You call repeatedly, but Dad does not answer.

» When Dad eventually answers the phone, the conversation is brief.

» Dad mistakes you for his brother or long-deceased father.

> » Reacquainting Dad to your identity takes more time than available.

> » You become frustrated with Dad canceling your visits.

> » You are worried about his health and well-being, and you wonder what is happening to him.

The reality of Dad's decline hits you on your visit because his home has changed significantly. It is disorderly for the first time since you have known him, with mail and bills stacked up. As you investigate deeper, you find some bills have been paid twice and others not paid at all. Checks from nine months ago are not cashed.

Dad appears thin. He has skinned knees and bruises on his arms and legs, but he denies falling. He walks very unsteadily, occasionally holding onto furniture that cannot hold his weight.

The neighbors notice your car and quickly greet you at Dad's door, conveying their concerns for your father's safety. They explain how he goes for long walks and is gone for hours; although he denies being lost, he is relieved when they walk him back home. The lawn, previously your dad's pride and joy, appears like a forest. You are relieved that Dad's car has not been driven, but you suspect that the keys are misplaced. You do not know how to handle the situation.

Where Do You Go? What Do You Do?

You call siblings, who are busy with their own lives, and they doubt that anything could be that bad. They explain how Dad recently seemed alert, remembered their birthday, and sent money; however, they realize that he had sent much more than the usual $50 gift. All agree that it is time for a family meeting at Dad's home to address his decline in memory.

The siblings convene. Dad denies that anything is wrong. He refuses to move from his home of thirty-five wonderful years or to have strangers in his home for assistance. The siblings all realize that something must be done, but they are fearful that it will be time-consuming and costly and that it will add stress to their already highly stressful lives. The stress overwhelms the children because of potential increased cost, time, frustration, and a complicated circumstance.

Who is responsible for the fact that Dad's decline was previously unnoticed? Blame shifts from one to another with each sibling describing their life as busier than the others, and all feel embarrassed and guilt-ridden about failing to recognize Dad's situation earlier. The tension, frustration, and guilt result in arguments more typical of school-aged children.

Usually, one sibling steps up and cares for the parent. During the first several months, the other siblings gladly call to see how things are going. Eventually, the first sibling wears down, giving another brave sibling a chance to take over. A year may pass before you find your sibling dropping off Mom or Dad at your doorstep. Now it is your turn.

You realize the impact that taking care of an aging parent has on your life. You realize what a difficult year it was for your brother or sister who stepped up first, dealing with the tribulations of caring for a parent with dementia. You begin to see the magnitude of the disease you are about to embrace, because dementia can be an invisible monster.

The Invisible Monster

Physical issues are visible and can be evaluated with concrete measurements. It is easy to quantify healing wounds, broken bones, and skin rashes. We may use X-rays or blood tests to help follow progress and confirm appropriate treatment.

What if the injury to the body is not something visible with X-rays or blood tests? What if the physical process of decline is invisible, despite devastating consequences? The invisible illness of memory loss or dementia occurs in the mind, and decline cannot be measured with tangible or visual calculations. Memory tests exist, but they are not precise. I refer to dementia as the *invisible monster* because it cannot be seen physically, and deterioration can be catastrophic.

Occasionally, we may forget things, names of people, or the location of our keys. Although such forgetfulness is normal, dementia is not about being forgetful. When forgetfulness becomes frequent and affects the daily routine, the person may be developing dementia. It is amazing how some people with dementia may recall facts from the past, such as a childhood address, names of friends not seen in twenty years, or a detailed sequence of random events that happened years ago.

Although we cannot see or measure the changes precisely, our mind may not be protected from the process of deterioration, even if we consume nutrient-dense foods and supplements that support brain function. As our parent's mind ages, he or she may begin to forget the little things, such as returning phone calls or paying the bills.

Memory decline gradually starts to impact their life consistently beyond basic daily events, with progressive disruption. Mom's forgetfulness surpasses beyond forgetting where she placed the keys or her purse. When the memory decline progresses, Mom may forget what she had for breakfast that morning or whether she ate breakfast. Dad cannot remember if he took a shower in the past several days.

Why does this progressive deterioration of the mind occur? Several factors may lead to this situation, including:

» blood pathways blocked by clots of blood in tiny vessels that feed the brain, more commonly known as a stroke;

» unexplained deterioration of brain tissue that hinders normal function and causes Alzheimer's dementia;

» other diseases of memory loss, such as Lewy Body Disease;

» chronic nutritional insufficiency, such as deficiencies of vitamin E, C, and B12.

No matter what label we place on the monster of dementia, we recognize that the brain is a body part that may deteriorate with aging or disease.

How can we best contend with the invisible monster of dementia? My successful approach to caring for people is not to focus on the "why" or "what kind," but to improve remaining function. An elder person without dementia may lose her eyesight and adjust to the world by using her other senses, such as touch, hearing, and intuition, to the best of her ability as she approaches the challenges of her surrounding environment. Similarly, an older person with dementia may increase social graces and simplify her environment to compensate for loss of memory.

People often wonder whether those who have dementia are aware of their condition. Mom or Dad with dementia is dealing with memory loss and is aware of her or his inabilities and declining condition. This awareness of an altered memory or perception is analogous to that caused by mind-altering medications or alcohol intoxication. A person who forgets or misplaces items, or who is overworked and fatigued, usually is aware of the forgetfulness.

However, as Mom ages, she may notice that she is not remembering some facts. Initially, she may laugh it off, attributing this to a transient lapse of memory. Mom may be in denial about her progressive memory loss. However, as memory lapses and mishaps occur, she may become aware that this problem is permanent. Mom may know that she is less able and more vulnerable, and she may experience anxiety or fear.

Mom may be embarrassed, feel stupid, and make efforts to hide or minimize the extent of her memory loss. This becomes her secret, and she perfects hiding her forgetfulness with simple social crutches. She stops calling you by name and refers to you as "honey," "sweetheart," and "darling." Nobody, including you, seems to have a clear identity or first name.

Where's My Wife?

A new resident, Harold, who had beginning stages of Alzheimer's dementia, moved into our assisted living community. His wife, Barbara, had been caring for him at home and was mentally and emotionally exhausted. She arranged for Harold to move in alone and planned to visit him as frequently as possible.

He could not remember his location or why he was in assisted living, and he constantly wondered about where his wife was located. Harold had no short-term memory. Although staff reminded him that he was staying at the assisted living community and that his wife would be coming to visit, a new conversation would occur every twenty minutes, with the same questions and answers. He wanted to be with his wife and go home where he remembered feeling safe.

Several days after he had moved to assisted living, Harold approached me at the front desk, repeating the same questions:

- » How do I get home?
- » Why am I here?
- » Where is my wife, Barbara?
- » When will I see her?

This time, I responded with questions. I asked him if he noticed that he sometimes forgot things. He sadly said, "Yes, I have Alzheimer's dementia." I asked him how he felt about this, and his response was that he was scared and felt unsafe. I asked him if he trusted his wife to make safe choices for him, and he responded, "Yes." I told him that Barbara had chosen this assisted living residence for him to stay safe while she was gone, and she would come back to visit.

Harold was aware that he would forget our entire conversation, so we wrote all this information on a piece of paper for him. He placed this paper in his shirt pocket. I asked him if he wanted me to show him his apartment, even though the directions were on the paper, and he said, "Yes." As we stood in the elevator together, Harold turned to me and said, "This Alzheimer's is a bummer."

He was truly aware of his situation. I put my arm around Harold and reassured him that we were in this together, and we would stay with him. Harold felt fearful and vulnerable in this new, unfamiliar environment of assisted living. Our job was to embrace Harold's memory loss and make him feel safe in his new home.

Most family members do not recognize the early stages of memory loss for a long time because symptoms of memory loss may be well hidden in casual conversation. My grandmother never called me by my given name; she referred to my siblings and me as "honey" or "sweetheart." It was not until my grandmother's memory loss progressed further that we became aware of her dementia and its severity.

Eventually, people find themselves in more serious situations, such as arriving at places without remembering how they got there. They quietly dismiss such an event and do not share the embarrassment. Morning walks become daylong walks with no memory of the way back or where the person lives. Sometimes a neighbor will direct an individual back home, or by chance, Dad eventually may recognize something familiar, hopefully his front door. All this is kept secret out of fear of being discovered, fearful of showing vulnerability in a world in which survival is hard enough without the added handicap of dementia. This fear drives a person to create behaviors to hide weakness of memory loss.

Advancing Dementia

As the dementia progresses and more things become unfamiliar, more situations are dangerous for Dad. He may resist anything that does not feel familiar or safe to him, even the most commonplace situations. A simple stream of water from the shower might feel unfamiliar and unsafe, and he may refuse to take showers. Unfamiliar people may be trying to encourage him to participate in unfamiliar activities. However, with memory loss, *most* activities have become unfamiliar.

In more extreme situations, Dad may feel under attack, and he may become combative, avoiding assistance with dressing or undressing. Adult children may become frustrated with the violence, being hit by Dad while they are trying to help him change his clothing. Dad with dementia is in a "fight or flight" survival mode and is reacting with out-of-control feelings because he does not recognize his environment. He is no longer familiar with the adult children or most daily situations. As a result, he may feel anger, anxiety, and depression.

It is important to help Mom or Dad feel safe, secure, and loved as she or he is losing the ability to recognize the familiar. It also is important that they feel needed and valued. It is most helpful that they are given positive feedback after completing small accomplishments, and not made to feel inadequate or stupid. This is all part of the recipe for successful care with dementia. As the caregiver, you can provide the little, caring things during the day that greatly help, such as:

»   holding Mom's hand,

»   telling her that she is loved and reminding her of her family that loves her,

»   providing familiar items from her home that she remembers,

» giving her tasks of importance that she can successfully complete,

» focusing on positive experiences from the past and present.

With repeated reminders, supportive conversations, and encouragement, Mom or Dad will experience more positive moments and, most importantly, feel loved.

Welcome to a New World

As we progress through life, we learn how to react to the physical world around us. We cry when we are traumatized. We learn about pain and how to avoid it. We learn about feelings of discomfort that result from heartbreak, physical injury, and even bad food. We also learn about the enjoyment of pleasure that results from love, great cuisine, and gentle touches.

We attach ourselves to the many experiences that give pleasure and learn how to best avoid pain. We can do this because of our awareness of our environment and the ability to think about personal interactions. However, in the person with dementia, the sensations may be present, but the ability of the mind to react is lost. As the mind deteriorates, the person loses the ability to process logic, reason, and learned cause and effect.

The most recent events are newest to the mind and more readily forgotten. The person with dementia does not remember simple recent daily events, such as where he or she was one hour ago or if a meal was eaten earlier in the day. Mom cannot remember what she did earlier that day or how she got dressed. The repeated long-term memories are more resistant to being forgotten, but they, too, become affected as dementia progresses.

In the more advanced stages of dementia, Dad does not remember his neighbors, address, or home state for the past eighty-four years. He may not remember exactly who you are. He may remember that you are someone familiar, and he may believe that a sibling or spouse is actually a son or daughter. As memory and logic deteriorate, Dad's perception of reality is transient, and he may experience his next thought without any recollection of previous thought.

After a thought enters Dad's mind, it becomes reality to him and difficult to convince him otherwise. He is comforted by the thought that he believes to be true in the present moment. He becomes attached to this thought and does not want to let go of it. This is one way that Dad's mind works abnormally because of dementia.

Three Men and a Memory

Dad's experience of living with dementia can be improved with a supportive approach. To illustrate such a situation, I recount an experience with three elderly residents of the assisted living community: Tom, Jim, and Frank. On a warm, sunny day, I arranged to go for a short, spontaneous walk with them. They seemed to know that they could not venture out by themselves because they would most likely not find their way back. After some discussion and confirmation that nothing else was occurring for them at that moment, they agreed to go.

Before departing, each man returned to his apartment several times: first for the correct cane, then for a sweater (even though it was eighty degrees outside), and finally for sunglasses or a hat. After walking just two blocks, they decided a rest was needed. We stopped at a medical building where there was a little coffee shop in the lobby. Each ordered drip coffee because lattes and cappuccinos were out of their comfort zone. As they sat and sipped their coffees, they had conversation among themselves.

I listened to each of the men as they recalled the details of their distant past. There was no conversation about recent events, including their present living situation and life. Recent memories were not included in the three elderly men's conversation because they were sketchy and unclear. Instead, the conversation reverted to the comfort of long-term memories, and they compared war stories from experiences earlier in their lives. The three men reflected on the details of these personal experiences with such apparent clarity, as if these events had just occurred the previous day. Two of the men had been in World War II, and the third man had been in the Korean War.

Tom, in his nineties, explained his version of being from Estonia and fighting on the "wrong" side. When the Germans occupied his area, he was recruited to work in the German Army intelligence. However, the German personnel discovered that he was originally from Estonia, and they were unhappy about this. One night, the Gestapo came for him, but he was tipped off and made a narrow escape. The two other war veterans were captivated by Tom's interesting near-capture experiences, and after noticing a stub on his left hand, they began to wonder how he had lost a finger.

Frank and Jim anticipated another heroic story about how Tom lost his finger, and they were amused to learn that the accident occurred when he was a child and his father was babysitting. All agreed that a father as a babysitter, in those days, was surely more dangerous than a war situation.

The stories and memories were recounted in conversation as if they had just recently happened. The situation, created with the men having conversation over coffee, embraced memories that were familiar and safe for them. Although the stories may have deviated in detail from the actual events, it was clear that the conversation helped make all three men feel that they had no memory problems at all.

CHAPTER 3

Deeper into Dementia

Defining the Stages

Clinicians may label Mom or Dad's dementia with a stage to define the severity of memory loss, categorize the problem, and concisely describe the patient's situation. However, disability of the mind is not easy to quantify because it is not something that can be seen or precisely measured. The tests for staging are done by observing the symptoms, which may vary at different times, and memory testing may be inaccurate.

There are several memory scales to help quantify dementia. Some scales calculate the level of dementia by assessing behavior, communication, delusions, and memory recall. Memory testing can be confusing, and different memory tests result in different numbered outcomes, some more simple than others. One memory test may describe dementia level at stage 3 on a scale of 3, but another may describe it at stage 7 on scale of 10.

Furthermore, test results do not help direct the appropriate approach for care, because the test may identify what Mom or Dad is experiencing only at the moment the test was administered. Symptoms of dementia may be worse or better at different times of the day. Therefore, it is more important to pay attention to the patterns of dementia symptoms to identify an effective approach for care.

Labeling dementia with a stage number also may limit care providers from exploring other care options available for patients at a specific level. Memory loss may be affected by the familiarity of the setting, which may affect the ability of a person to adapt. When Mom or Dad has difficulty adapting to the environment, dementia may seem more pronounced, and the care may require more adjustments and supports.

It may not be helpful to label dementia with a stage because a minor change of circumstances can make dementia symptoms seem more or less pronounced. The perceived stage of dementia can change for reasons other than environment. Dementia can seem more severe because of depression, changes in medication, or infection. The level of dementia can seem more advanced when the care setting is inappropriate. Mom's impairment may seem worse than it was previously, even if the severity of dementia has not deteriorated, because she may be withdrawn from boredom.

"I Don't Belong Here"

An inappropriate care setting may affect the level of dementia. Several years ago, a family requested that I evaluate their mother, Violet, for placement in the assisted living community. They described Violet as nonverbal, withdrawn, and wanting to escape from her present community. Violet had stopped eating. She had recently been moved to a locked area with other patients who had more advanced dementia, and she was not allowed to leave the area by herself.

When I went to evaluate Violet, she was in her new apartment in the gated area. Other residents of this area required a higher level of care, could not participate in simple conversations, and needed total care for dressing, bathing, and eating. I read Violet's chart, spoke with staff, and visited her apartment. She was lying in bed, and she seemed very sad and alone. She felt helpless because this environment was inappropriate for her cognitive level, and this caused her to retreat to the solitude of her bed.

Violet's room was dark because the lights were off and shades were pulled closed. When I asked her if I could sit next to her, she seemed happy to have company, and she agreed. As I sat beside Violet on her bed, she did not look up at me or make any eye contact. I spoke with her and asked questions but received only nods or shakes of her head in return. Violet understood me, but I felt a barrier between us because she did not engage in conversation. The barrier was her sadness.

Violet's level of dementia was difficult to assess because it was overshadowed by her extreme sadness that limited communication. I gave her a memory test, and she scored a perfect 30/30. This confirmed that she had minimal memory loss and did not have extreme dementia, but depression. She knew that she was not confused and now seemed hopeful that this was finally recognized.

Violet had been misplaced in a high-dementia area, but she had little memory loss. Furthermore, the staff had assumed that her lack of interaction was from severe dementia, and they did not recognize that it had been caused by depression. She was experiencing very little meaningful interaction with other residents, who had advanced memory loss and behavioral issues. Her situation had seemed hopeless, and she had become so severely depressed that she became immobilized in bed. The staff had rarely spoken to Violet because she did not respond. As her depression became worse, she stopped eating, and the staff had assumed that Violet was entering a stage of late or advanced dementia.

Later in our conversation, Violet was able to look me in the eyes, and I asked her if she would approve a move to another care community. With tears in her eyes, she answered with a simple and soft, "Yes." I felt that she trusted me, and she knew that I could help her.

The next day, Violet was transferred to the assisted living community where I was working. By simply changing to a more stimulating environment, she blossomed. She began to interact with higher functioning people and had marked improvements in her abilities. She became more interactive, participatory, and engaged in her environment. She rarely stayed in her apartment, and she preferred to eat in the main dining room, participate in activities, socialize, or simply enjoy the day with her million-dollar smile.

Violet's story is an example of how an inappropriate environment can cause further decline, and how improvement may be noted in a more appropriate environment of care. She had appeared to have more advanced dementia because she was depressed. She had been labeled by staff as having an incorrect stage of dementia, and this had resulted in an inaccurate care plan and further decline. However, this situation improved, and a more stimulating environment seemed to awaken "sleeping brain cells."

"State of Mind" Is State of Health

If Mom or Dad feel empowered, they will act stronger. If sad, they will likely disengage and display a lower level of functioning. My approach to dementia is to create a setting with the most stimulating situations possible. This provides people with the opportunity to connect with their higher level of interaction and to "rise to the occasion." This concept disregards the negative effect of labeling the stages of dementia. By addressing the unique symptoms of each individual, we enable them to reach their highest potential.

The will to live is driven by a connection with "purpose." If there is purpose, there is an increased desire to participate. Purpose can lead to increased happiness and willingness to participate in other aspects of daily life. People are more willing to eat well at meals and become more physically active, and this is important to maintain and improve health.

It is difficult to disregard the advice of well-meaning experts who limit the possibilities for Dad with dementia by classifying him at a stage level. The stage category may create a self-fulfilling, limiting prophesy of what staff and families believe he cannot do. This may result in people giving up, instead of pushing, experimenting, and testing what he can excel at doing or improving. It is healthier for Mom to look beyond categorized perceived limits of what she can do and explore the limits of what may seem impossible. A staging is sometimes a diagnosis that will limit direction of care by causing people to give up trying to improve. Given the opportunity, even with the label of Alzheimer's disease, your mom may surprise you with abilities you did not believe were present.

Memory loss can be staged in three general categories:

» mild

» moderate

» severe

Mild Memory Loss

Mild memory loss includes forgetting events of the day, which is more than simply misplacing the car keys or purse. Forgetting becomes a frequent, daily occurrence that becomes disruptive to daily life. It becomes routine to forget that the bills have been paid and to pay them several times. The person becomes an easy target for any scam artist, because he or she is still in control of financial matters but cannot manage them properly. Mom or Dad might leave the stove on or wear the same outfit each day. He or she repeatedly calls family because the previous call, the same day, has been forgotten.

People with mild memory loss function at a higher level than those with moderate or severe memory loss, but the care is difficult. Mom and Dad with mild memory loss may be resistant to changing their situation. They refuse help from others to correct miscalculations in bills and with the general tasks of the day. They may be driving a car, but they forget where they are going, and they never make it to the family event at the adult children's homes. Dad may stop his car to fill up with gas, only to find that the gas tank is already full. His mind is overloaded and stressed from many thoughts of trying to identify his surroundings, so his reaction time while driving is delayed. Adult children must ensure safety and prevent Dad from driving, but his denial of memory loss makes him resist having the car taken away. People deny the fact that mild memory loss impairs driving, and this is analogous to the lack of awareness of people who are intoxicated with alcohol that they are unsafe to drive home.

Dad may be aware of losing his memory, and he may be frustrated and angry with the mistakes made while driving. However, he hopes that he will be back to normal the next time he drives. In his denial, he does not accept any help from others when failing, and this is a warning sign that his memory decline is truly taking place. With mild memory loss, people usually believe that all is well and that life will continue without change.

With mild stages of dementia, Mom may be in denial and attempt to maintain the illusion that her memory is normal. As time progresses, memory lapses recur, and it becomes more difficult to fool others into believing that she is completely aware and functional. The adult children may get professional help from a doctor or lawyer to address the reality of memory loss, but occasionally these professionals are fooled by Mom or Dad's alert times and may not recognize the extent of memory loss and dangers with dementia. These professionals may decline to limit Mom from handling her own affairs or change her power of attorney. In an effort to retain her decision-making power over financial matters, Mom may seek out her own attorney to resist her children's efforts to gain control. An attorney that Mom hires may only hear her altered and very believable story of being a victim of her greedy children who want her money.

Children sometimes find themselves in lengthy legal battles to gain control of Mom's financial affairs for her protection. During these legal battles, it is unfortunate for the adult children that Mom seems to communicate and remember better than usual, and she may give the impression that she is fine when speaking with her attorney.

Phoebe's Story

At eighty-two years old, Phoebe still had a dry sense of humor. Friends and family enjoyed her unique personality traits, even after she had developed spotty memory loss from minor strokes. Strangers were entertained by her ability to keep up with a conversation and cleverly sum things up with a witty or sassy comment. These strangers did not know that Phoebe lived at an assisted living community and was unable to manage at home independently. With limited interactions with strangers, Phoebe could convince them that she was of sound mind and able to care for and make decisions for herself.

However, Phoebe also suffered from delusions and occasional paranoid thoughts that caused her to make poor decisions and choices. She thought that her daughter was stealing from her. She did not remember requesting that the painting on the wall be removed; later, she noticed that the painting was missing from her wall and believed that it was stolen. She spent some evenings cutting up her pillows, and the feathers from the pillows flew everywhere and caused her to slip and fall. When asked why she cut up her pillows, she appeared puzzled, unable to figure out what had happened. She cleverly responded, "The feathers needed fresh air." Although her knives and scissors were removed from her apartment, she coerced another resident to lend her a different pair of scissors or a knife. As a result of these delusions and paranoid thoughts, she sometimes injured herself or created a mess in her apartment that could have harmed her.

Phoebe's daughter, Carrie, noticed trouble after Phoebe went on outings or excursions to the bank. At first, Phoebe made small cash withdrawals for shopping. However, on one occasion, she had delusions and became paranoid, thinking that someone could get into her account. She closed her bank account and opened another. The bank tellers loved her and became familiar with her, all the time believing she was in her right mind.

Carrie wrote a check for her mother's expenses but found that the account was closed and there were no funds available. Phoebe began having delusions that Carrie was stealing her money and refused to give her signing authority on her new bank account. Carrie's attempts to stop Phoebe's banking transactions were ignored by the bank, because the tellers believed that Phoebe was being swindled by her greedy daughter. It took several months, working with doctors and lawyers, to get Phoebe's bank accounts under Carrie's safe supervision.

When adult children step in to assist Mom or Dad, they can enter a situation characterized by:

» resistance,

» threats and alienation,

» emotional stress,

» time consumption,

» financial duress.

These are common experiences that adult children endure when helping a parent with mild memory loss. Nevertheless, the support from adult children who take over the parent's affairs is essential for safety and well-being. It may be necessary at this early stage of memory loss to have Mom or Dad placed in a care environment where they will receive appropriate care.

Many times, Mom or Dad may have resistance to releasing control of the decisions about finances and care to their children, and this can result in Mom or Dad staying alone in their home longer. Eventually, a catastrophic event may occur when Mom goes for a walk and becomes lost or has a fall that leads to hospitalization, and this may catalyze movement into an assisted care situation.

This initial exposure to mild dementia is a new problem for the family. Adult children must learn how to handle each new forgetful situation and realize that more experiences are just around the corner. However, adult children have many safe options to care for Mom or Dad with mild dementia. Increased monitoring may be accomplished with environmental changes. These include:

» moving Mom or Dad into the child's home;

» hiring help in Mom or Dad's own home;

» placing Mom or Dad in a care environment, such as an assisted living or group home.

Initially, the least disruptive and simplest change usually is to hire assistance for them in their home. This may avoid the stress and increased confusion of changing living environments.

The daily challenges of mild dementia may be too difficult to have Mom or Dad move in with their adult children. Many adult children choose not to upset their family's environment, and they avoid having a parent move in. It usually is a better choice for everyone to provide care elsewhere than the adult children's home, because it usually is a huge stress to provide the constant monitoring needed when living with the family.

The better alternative is to have Mom or Dad cared for in another care environment. This option avoids disruption of family life and provides experts to care for Mom or Dad. However, financial cost is a major factor with the assisted living or group home environments and usually is the main deterrent to obtaining this kind of care, because not all families can afford this expense.

When Mom and Dad are placed in a more monitored, safe environment with less to manage and less stress, they usually improve in many ways. They may stop stumbling and falling because the care environment provides care support. Care staff may remind Dad to use the walker, to drink water and avoid episodes of dehydration and dizziness, and to correctly manage his medications. Mom and Dad may sleep better at night after healthy evening meals, and they may find comfort because others are doing chores for them.

With increased basic care in the new environment, Mom or Dad can be more functional and alert. After they notice improvement in the alternative care environment, they may feel better or cured, and they may insist on returning home. However, returning home to the less monitored environment may create the same situation they experienced previously. It may be an ongoing struggle to convince Mom or Dad to remain in the more monitored care situation for her or his own well-being.

In the early period, when Mom has mild memory loss and is living away from her long-term home in the alternative care environment of the assisted living or group home, she may believe that she is managing her own health-care and financial affairs. It is important to support Mom so she believes that she is still managing these aspects of her life, because this is what she has done since childhood. It is traumatic for Mom and Dad to lose lifelong responsibilities, and it is difficult for them to accept or understand that they are no longer capable of self-care.

Life Is a Puzzle

People with mild dementia may have difficulties with problem solving. Laura and Debra, two residents of an assisted living community, were sitting together having a casual conversation about the day's events. Suddenly, Laura became panicked because she realized that she had not been to the bank, and she could not remember when she last went to the bank. However, Laura had lived at the assisted living community for nine months and had not done her own banking since she moved in.

Debra said that she thought it made perfect sense for Laura to go to the bank. Debra asked Laura where she did her banking, and after pausing to think, Laura replied, "I don't remember! Where do you do your banking?" Debra seemed surprised that Laura could not remember where she did her banking. Then Debra realized that she had the same problem and said, "I can't remember." Debra concluded that maybe she did not need to go to the bank because she could not remember which bank she used.

As Debra continued to ponder her present situation, she turned to Laura and inquired, "What town are we in?" Laura was very resourceful at filling in the blanks for things she could not remember, and she quickly responded with the correct name of the town. Debra was relieved to know what town they were in but seemed confused that Laura knew the town but not the name of her bank. Debra asked Laura how she was so sure about the town. Laura turned and looked out the window at a parked van that had the assisted living advertisement and address. She replied, "Well, it says the town right there on the bus."

This conversation is a typical example of how Mom and Dad with early dementia may have trouble remembering daily details, such as names or places, and how they use cues from their surroundings to assist their memory. They may not remember routine tasks from the past, such as banking, but problem solving will bring about a conclusion that will comfort them. The problem-solving tactics of people with mild dementia may cause them to believe they still can manage safely on their own, despite the observations of the family.

Home on the Ranch

Leo, an eighty-year-old retired businessman, lived alone on his large ranch for thirty years. He took care of his property, which included many acres, horses, and a barn. He hired help to maintain the ranch and assist with the care of the horses, but he saw no need for assistance with his own care.

His two children, Nora and Cory, met with me at the assisted living residence. They had recently visited their father and found him lying on the floor in his house, unable to get up. He could not remember how long he had been lying there. This had not been the first time that Nora had come to his home and found that Leo had hurt himself. Leo previously had excuses for what had happened and refused to have anyone come to check or care for him in his home.

Nora noticed that Leo had lost weight and probably was not eating enough. The refrigerator and the trash were empty, and frozen foods in the freezer had not been used. Nora and her brother, Cory, took Leo to the hospital where Leo was diagnosed with a broken right arm. The hospital staff showed Nora and Cory many bruises and other injuries that Leo had received, probably from other falls in the home while on his own.

Nora and Cory understood that Leo needed care. They could not care for Leo in their home, so they chose an assisted living option for him. The hospital sent Leo for a short stay at a nursing home to recover from his injuries before entering the assisted living community. Leo arrived at the assisted living environment in a wheelchair because his earlier injuries from falls made him very unsteady and weak.

Leo was in the mild stages of dementia, but he maintained his stubborn and domineering personality that had made it difficult for Nora and Cory to change his living situation. He had previously controlled every aspect of his life, and he had dominated his children. Therefore, he was adamant that he was perfectly fine living on his own and managing his own affairs. Nevertheless, Leo initially came to our community willingly because he was anxious to leave the confining and rigid routines of the nursing home. His initial plan was to stay at the assisted living community just long enough to regain his strength so he could discard his wheelchair and resume walking, and he would then return home to his ranch to live alone.

Nora and Cory wanted Leo to stay at the assisted living community because they knew he was not competent to live safely on his own. They hoped that he would become accustomed to the place and like it. They knew that Leo would receive the proper care and restore his health in an environment with assistance. Fortunately, Nora and Cory had previously established power of attorney for health care and finances because Leo's physicians had recommended this precaution.

Leo recovered quickly in the assisted living community because he had the proper support for recovery in this care setting. He discarded the wheelchair and was walking with a cane within a few weeks. He regained the ability to dress and shower independently. The community provided Leo with the needed assistance to safely carry out daily functions, but without this type of supportive care, Leo would likely fall again. Unfortunately, Leo believed that he was ready to return to his prior home environment, and he demanded power of attorney status from his children, wanting control as primary decision maker for his affairs.

Leo was in denial about his forgetfulness and not aware of his inability to manage his personal care and finances outside the assisted living setting. Nora and Cory continued the struggle with Leo's mild dementia, but Leo began to contact lawyers and physicians to support his efforts to return home. Leo also began to call taxis to take him home. The taxi drivers, not aware of Leo's disabilities, found him very believable until a staff member corrected the situation.

Leo resumed his controlling tactics and domineering ways with his children, threatening that they would be removed from his will if they did not comply with his wishes. Nora and Cory were emotionally exhausted from calls to lawyers and other professionals to dispute Leo's orders. They were tired of arguing with Leo to manage his situation in his best interests. Leo eventually prevailed because of one physician's support, and he returned home.

Nora contacted us six months later because the situation had worsened, and staff at the ranch had taken advantage of Leo financially. Leo was able to problem solve and put enough cues together that would get him one step further in trouble. He believed that the staff at the ranch would help him remember things, enabling him to stay there safely. He decided to marry one of the female staff members to ensure that she would continue taking care of him. Nora was outraged when she found the staff member wearing her deceased mother's engagement ring.

The legal battle continued. Despite his mild dementia, Leo had enough problem-solving tactics to convince doctors and lawyers that he was able to make decisions about his finances and was safe at his ranch. Unfortunately, he was making desperate decisions in a false reality of dementia to enable him to stay at home.

Moderate Memory Loss

Moderate memory loss is more noticeable than mild memory loss. With moderate memory loss, people see the effects of forgetfulness that cannot be hidden. Falls are routine, people dress themselves inappropriately, wearing bras on the outside or donning three shirts. It becomes difficult to learn anything new in the living environment, and only long-term events remain embedded in the memory bank.

The only hope of accomplishing a new task independently is to have many repetitive experiences, so the event becomes an ingrained, automatic pattern of behavior without conscious thought processes. With moderate dementia, learning a new task that changes even small events of Mom or Dad's day can take several weeks to become routine. It may require six weeks or longer to become acclimated to major changes, such as relocation. Short-term memory is lost, and Mom repeats the same statements within minutes. Every day is a new experience because Dad does not remember prior days. It is helpful for the assisted living community to take photographs of events and activities to help him remember.

Memories of the past may remain clear, including details of names and dates. This can be refreshing and comforting. Families and caregivers may focus on past memories because the spark of life burns brightly inside Mom or Dad when they talk about events that are clear and familiar to them. The moderate stage typically is easier for the family to manage than the mild stage. Mom and Dad may not argue about having control of the finances because they are unaware that this issue exists. They may not insist on going home because they are confused about where home is located, and they may recall a childhood home but have no recollection of homes in their adult years. There may be no struggles about relinquishing the power of attorney, calling taxis, or needing friends to transport them home.

Speak My Way

Roslyn was nonverbal and had moderate memory loss when she entered the assisted living setting. When she spoke, she would string just enough key words together to get her message across. During the months that Roslyn's dementia progressed, she stopped using words altogether and resorted simply to pointing to what she desired.

One day, I entered the higher care area where she resided. A new staff member from the Philippines was caring for Roslyn for the first time, unaware that Roslyn was totally nonverbal. The caregiver knew that Roslyn was from the Philippines and spoke to her in her native language, assuming Roslyn would understand. To my amazement, Roslyn responded back in her native tongue, speaking in paragraphs in what seemed to be an intense conversation with the new staff member.

Watching these two people speak in a common language gave the impression that Roslyn did not have dementia at all, so I asked the staff caregiver what Roslyn was saying. She explained that Roslyn was making perfect sense and was telling her about where she was from and about her family. Roslyn had forgotten the English that she had learned as an adult. In her moderate stage of dementia, she could only remember her native language. Communicating in her native language enabled Roslyn to reminisce about past events and revive an important interest. With this newly found communication, Roslyn was able to regain that spark of life that had been lost.

Total Care

Moderate to severe memory loss frequently requires total care. Dressing, bathing, and eating may not occur without significant hands-on assistance. This may be physically exhausting for staff that provide this level of assistance, and it may be emotionally difficult for the family to see Dad needing this much care. In this late stage of dementia, medications to control behavior are frequently prescribed for Dad because he may not respond to reason and has little or no control over his emotions. Behaviors may be random and without logical purpose. Thoughts may be spontaneous, and statements may not make any sense.

Adult children no longer recognize Dad as the same person he was previously. Dad may not recognize family members. One wife of a resident was disturbed that her husband frequently asked her the whereabouts of his wife and family. She responded that she was Emily, his wife, but he refused to believe her. The husband had only long-term memories of Emily when she was younger, possibly in her forties, and did not recognize his wife, now in her eighties. Emily brought family photographs, and her husband pointed to a picture of her in her younger years and said, "That's my wife."

Severe Memory Loss

Advanced stages of dementia require more of an effort from the caregiver to provide support in every aspect of humanity and dignity for Mom or Dad. Mom may not initiate any aspect of care needed. Dad may urinate in a drinking fountain, sink, plant, or corner, or may defecate in his clothing or on the carpet.

When Dad's condition declines to a minimal level of functioning and dignity, many families will have discussions with the physician about the handling of aggressive medical support. The adult children may subtly view Dad as his former self, and they may feel that he is still very much alive. The family reaches out and embraces these moments because this provides the fuel for their supporting Dad emotionally. With severe memory loss, Dad's internal desire to live will carry him through another day. Until Dad loses that will to live, it is important to stand by him and continue to support his efforts in health as best as possible. In this extreme situation of total care for physical and mental support, staff caregivers should do everything to make Dad's life experience as wonderful and meaningful as possible.

The Hidden Handicap

When Mom was younger, with a strong mind and good physical health, she was able to do almost anything. She was prepared to tackle the daily routine with ease. From the time she woke up, she could independently and effortlessly perform the daily tasks of bathing, dressing, and preparing her meals.

She completed the daily tasks with little thought or effort. Eventually, as her mind began to fail, she became challenged by not remembering the most basic things. She now had the handicap of dementia. Everything became a challenge to complete because nothing was remembered as routine. Dementia limited her abilities to perform basic tasks of the day.

Handicaps exist in many forms. Some are easily seen, such as a physical handicap. However, a mental or emotional disability may be less obvious to detect in the early stages. Dementia is a handicap that develops late in life because of the mind's deterioration, and it is one of the greatest handicaps to affect health care. Unfortunately, it is not aggressively referred to as a handicap or treated as such, because this handicap is a common end result of life for the older person. Dementia is approached by the medical community as a disease.

Any type of handicap will affect individuals differently and to varying degrees. Some people with an amputation are very limited in their daily activities, but others with the same amputation may compete in sports and challenge the day, rather than have the day challenge them.

When a person has a physical handicap, either temporary or permanent (such as a broken leg or spinal injury), he adjusts to his new world of decreased mobility by using assistive devices, such as crutches, canes, or wheelchairs. With a physical handicap, adjustments needed to assist Mom are concrete and easy to see. However, dementia is not a visible disability, and it may be difficult to make the needed adjustments to help Mom. In addition, the adjustments Mom needs for assistance with dementia may be difficult to identify because her symptoms and behaviors can be inconsistent.

Instead of canes, walkers, crutches, or wheelchairs, the dementia handicap may be assisted with memory aids, such as reminder notes, or medications to improve memory. Although physical handicaps are immediately apparent from the time of occurrence, dementia requires studying Mom's behavioral patterns and then making adjustments.

With all types of dementia, we must gauge the extent of Mom's dementia handicap by examining the decrease in her abilities, including communication, and changes in her behavior.

What Kind of Dementia Is It, Anyway?

There are several different causes of dementia that result in different types of behavioral patterns. It is helpful to have a correct diagnosis of the cause, to help with the approach of dealing with the memory deficit. In dementia that is caused by disease, such as Alzheimer's, Parkinson's, or Lewy Body disease, there may be a gradual and predictable decline. In dementia caused by vascular changes resulting from a stroke, blood flow is limited to certain areas of the brain; memory or physical changes may be random, and short-term memory may not be affected, but it may be difficult to solve the problem of how to proceed with a simple task.

Dementia also may be caused by age-related memory loss or other medical conditions, such as infection, dehydration, or vitamin B12 deficiency. It is important to notice a change in behavior, such as increased memory loss or behavioral problems. Such a change may not be the normal progression of Mom or

Dad's dementia, but rather, it may occur because of the onset of a treatable additional illness. Toxic exposure to mold or a chemical is a treatable illness that may mimic symptoms of dementia. In some patients, dementia could be entirely from the effects of this toxic exposure, and not from Alzheimer's disease. When symptoms of dementia are caused by exposure to chemicals or other toxic environmental factors, normal memory can return after the body is clear of these substances. Mental or emotional disorders and improper medication management can cause Mom or Dad to experience disorientation, and these symptoms may appear similar to dementia symptoms. Therefore, it is very important to explore the cause of memory loss with a qualified doctor so it can be corrected and reversed.

Richard's Battle with Mold

Richard, an eighty-three-year-old retired pilot, had a mistaken diagnosis of Alzheimer's dementia. He was in the hospital, and his family requested that I visit him for an evaluation for acceptance to our assisted living center. Richard was unable to remember how he came to the hospital, and he had moderate memory loss. He had fresh cuts and bruises on his legs and arms, but he could not explain how they developed.

Richard had been living at home with his wife, Helen, who described him as becoming more confused during the past year. He was occasionally out of control and combative. One morning, Helen could not find Richard, but after searching their large home, she eventually found him wedged between a wall and the refrigerator. Richard's adult children were called to the home to help Helen free Richard from this position and take him to the hospital. The adult children felt that Helen could no longer care for him safely and suggested that he be placed in an assisted living center directly after discharge from the hospital.

After his hospitalization, Richard was admitted to the higher care section of the assisted living community. He had significant memory loss, scoring only five points (out of a maximum of thirty points) on a memory test. He was unable to follow directions, walk, or feed himself.

During the following year, Richard's condition improved gradually. He was able to remember things, albeit slowly. He improved physically and was able to walk, dress independently, and eat by himself. He eventually was transferred to the area of the assisted living center where less care was required. The memory test was repeated, and he had a normal score of thirty points.

The family transferred Richard to a group home soon after his full recovery, but doctors initially were unable to explain his recovery and return to good health. Several years later, the family told me that they discovered that his home had been infested with black mold, which had caused his state of moderate to severe dementia. After he had been removed from this toxic mold environment, his body was cleared of the effects of the mold, and he recovered.

Wrong Medications

The wrong medications may cause a condition of extreme anxiety, including symptoms of dementia and new behavioral problems.

Terri and Joseph had been married for sixty-five years. They lived in an assisted living home that provided basic services without nursing care. During the previous three months, Terri had become confused, emotional, and so anxious that she could not complete even the simplest task.

The assisted living home requested that they move because of this change in Terri's condition. Although Terri was not disruptive to the assisted living community, they were unable to provide care for her with her new symptoms. She needed help to bathe, get dressed, and take her medications. When she was anxious, she walked continually and could not sleep at night. Terri's anxiety became so intense that she could not sit, eat, or sleep. She was unable to remember from minute to minute, and she asked the same questions repeatedly. Joseph was emotionally and physically exhausted, and he could not take care of her.

Terri's primary doctor was perplexed about the cause of her escalated anxiety and forgetfulness. However, he discovered that Terri had recently been seen at the hospital for an infection, and the hospital doctor had changed her medication. These medication changes were in addition to other changes made in recent months. It was difficult to decipher which medication changes might have been causing adverse reactions of anxiety.

Terri was admitted for a short stay in a mental health hospital to determine which medications were appropriate for her. In the hospital setting, the doctors monitored Terri's reaction to the medications prescribed for her anxiety, and she was placed on medications that correctly addressed her anxiety disorder. They also stopped the other medications that had possibly given her the undesirable adverse effects of anxiety.

Terri's health improved to her condition from six months earlier, and she was discharged back to the assisted living community. Her anxiety was successfully treated with medication management, and her memory improved.

CHAPTER 4

Early Tactics of Caring

In the Beginning, We Try It at Home

As Dad declines in physical abilities and memory loss progresses, many adult children attempt to care for him at home. The goal may be to keep him home with family members who love him devotedly and care for him properly. However, many adult children cannot stay at home full-time because of jobs, chores, and unexpected time away.

Sometimes a family member may be at home most of the day to assist Dad with meals, bathing, daily walks, and changing clothes when he does not make it to the bathroom in time. Although there may be times when nobody is at home to assist or supervise Dad, there may be a window of time when he can stay at home, provided that certain strategies are in place for success. To tackle the goal of basic safety and care in the home while adult children are away, there are three general areas that families must address:

» nutritional needs and meals

» physical-care needs

» safety precautions during activities

Meals

Meal preparation can be an easy task to accomplish because there are many prepared or easy-to-fix options in grocery stores. For hot meals, there are community-based programs that can deliver a meal to the home. The key principle is to keep it simple, using written directions and reminders for Dad that are in his constant sight as much as possible.

A routine for acquiring and preparing meals is essential for success. Although his memory may be limited, patterns of behavior and familiar routines may help him with meals.

Tips to Consider:

1. **Written instructions** should be in large, clear print and placed in the same location each day. The kitchen counter is a good place because Dad will see the note when he enters the kitchen to get something to eat.

2. **Keep it simple.** Place prepared plates of food in the refrigerator and label these plates. Use clear wrap, not foil, so Dad can see what is on the plate. It is simpler if the food can be eaten unheated. If the food must be heated, always label the microwave with an arrow or sticker to identify the correct button. Frozen foods are simple; open the box and label it, so it is ready in the freezer.

3. **Snacks and nutritional drinks** can be placed in clear view on the counter. Dad will want a snack and will open the first thing he sees.

Physical Care

Physical care for Dad in the home includes walking with him from one place to another, engaging him in an entertaining activity, or helping with hygiene as needed. In the home environment, Dad is kept engaged by participating in enjoyable activities. Dad may attempt to do things for himself beyond his present abilities, so it is best to provide items that he enjoys nearby.

His home space can be arranged by having the bathroom close to his television, favorite reading materials, desk, favorite chair, and bed. Assistance with physical aspects of hygiene can be organized around the adult children's work schedule. In the evening, he can be helped with a change in clothing and a basic shave. It may help to have a care agency assist with Dad's shower care twice per week. It is important for Dad to have a telephone nearby so he can call without having to get up, and the walker or cane should be next to him before he is left alone.

Safety

Safety is an important aspect of planning for Dad's needs while the adult children are away. Karen was unsuccessful in maintaining a safe environment for her father, Bill. Bill was in the early stages of dementia and not aware of his limitations. He had been the "fix-it guy" for his family throughout his entire life and felt compelled to continue with this activity. He was not willing to accept the reality that it was now unsafe to do so. He insisted on fixing things while she was gone and attempted to secure the gutters to the side of the roof. When Karen returned from her eight- to ten-hour workday, she found sharp utensils on the carpet and the water running in the bathroom sink; the ladder had been dragged from the garage and was leaning crookedly on the side of the house.

A successful approach to the problem of keeping Dad safe at home when alone or unattended requires imagination and creativity. Appropriate activities will keep Dad busy, mentally engaged, and stimulated. Sometimes the activities set up for the day include television and audio books, but problems may arise when Dad cannot start the audio, video, or television.

Some helpful tips include:

» Leave the television tuned to his favorite channel.

» Always have the DVD or audio books ready to start with just one button to press.

» Keep books of crossword puzzles or trivia on the table in plain view.

» If Dad loves his desk and has a history of paying bills, he may be left with a stack of bills to sort or write out. One strategy is to have an expired or closed account left with him to write out all the checks, with envelopes addressed to a post-office box address that belongs to an adult child.

Keeping the environment at home physically safe essentially means "child-proofing" an environment for a big person.

Tips for adult-proofing a home for the elderly include:

1. **Turn off the water** in sinks and bathtubs while he is left alone.
2. **Lock away all ladders, chemicals, and cleaning agents**.
3. **Lock away all knives** other than dinner knives.
4. **Disable all power tools and the lawn mower**.
5. **Provide a walker** if he is unsteady on his feet.
6. **Build a ramp** for the stairs.

Although it will be difficult to keep Dad at home with memory loss and physical-care needs, it can be done successfully on a temporary or permanent basis. When creative efforts fail, Dad may be placed outside the home in an alternative care environment, such as a group adult home or assisted living community. The change to a new home requires some tactics to encourage Dad to move and also involves a process of adjustment.

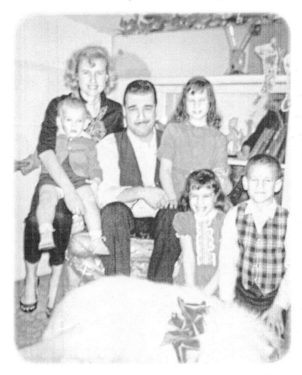

Home Is Where the Heart Is

People with dementia may remember only the most important memories, and for many, these memories involve the home. All they want to do is to return home. Home is a very meaningful place because it provides love, security, and safety. It is a place of familiarity and comfort. The nurturing home environment is where children develop and grow emotionally and physically to adulthood. Children are raised by parents who use patterns of nurturing learned from the grandparents and other family members. Ideally, the generations are connected with memories of love and safety at home.

Although the home environment may not always be pleasant or filled with fond memories, it is an important influence on a person's development. Even in the worst environments of childhood experiences, there may be a strong attachment to the family and home setting where some aspects of bonding occurred.

The home also is a place to collect and maintain the tangible reminders of life's experiences and memories. Many people place a high importance on their home. They spend their resources and time transforming their home to a place of desired comfort. The home becomes the centerpiece for many people, a "safety net" for them and their family. These valued feelings of home are remembered in the aging parent's core memory, and Mom and Dad have had a life's journey in creating these attachments to the home. Aging parents with dementia and memory loss show their attachment to home in several ways.

"Where Are You From?"

Hazel, a resident in our assisted living community, had very limited short-term memory. She used to repeatedly ask the same question about a person's home. As the person responded to her question, she repeated the same question, as if it had not been previously asked or answered just minutes ago.

With her limited conversation abilities, Hazel used to focus on the location and origin of a person's home, because this was her most valued subject. Hazel used to ask people, "Where are you from?" or "Where do you live?" People initially valued the subject of conversation, but unless they too had extensive memory loss, they had difficulty answering this question repeatedly.

The answer to Hazel's question seemed different for people of different generations. Many people from the baby boomer or younger generations may have moved from their childhood home for college, work, or adventure. They may reflect on the place in the recent past where they are "from" or where they consider as "home." Hazel valued home as the foundation, the place where all the basic family activities occurred. For Hazel, home was in Chicago, far from her current location because her adult children moved her to Seattle two years earlier. In Hazel's mind, Chicago remained the place she was "from" because it was the place she valued as home for much of her life.

In contrast with their adult children, many elderly people may not have moved far from their first home. Dad's generation did not move much, and his current living place may be where he had lived for much of his life, perhaps forty years or more. This is the place where Dad raised his family, enjoyed years of holiday celebrations, and threw a football with the grandchildren. Home for Dad is a place where many long-term patterns of behavior developed. There are very strong emotional attachments and behavior patterns referred to as "home" that are significant when addressing Dad's care in his elderly state with memory loss.

Heading for the Barn

Elderly residents routinely verbalize that they want to live at home. Although they may not know where home is located, because of memory decline, they know that it is a good place to be, and home is where they want to go. Home is usually the destination for Dad with dementia because he is seeking this secure place.

Behaviors such as trying to leave and go "home" may occur even when Dad has lived at his present home for many years. He may have a sense of home from his childhood and long-term memory that does not match the home he lives in presently.

Dad may be confused because of his memory loss, but he frequently has a very clear perception of which place is home. At some time, he may say that he wants to go home. This may occur regardless of his wonderful present situation in the adult children's home or the assisted living environment. Adult children should not be surprised if he frequently verbalizes that he wants to go home.

Dad may not adjust to considering another place as home, such as the adult children's home, alterative group home, or assisted living community. These environments may not replace the life patterns and conditions that qualify as his home from past memory. Although he may feel safe in his present care environment, it is not the same feeling of safety and love that he may feel from his past.

Dad may repeat that he wants to go home, and this may put tremendous guilt and stress on adult children or other family members who have placed their parent or spouse in care environments other than their own home. However, his ongoing statements of desire for his version of home should not be the reason to remove him from this environment where he is receiving needed care. This is best managed by using some techniques of guidance to help Dad avoid trying to leave this place of safety and care.

"Elopement" is the attempt of a person with dementia to leave the assisted living environment, a frequent behavior that is difficult to manage. This term is used in elderly health care to describe the behavior of leaving the care environment without staff or family consent when the person is unable to leave safely on his own.

Usually, a power of attorney is legally in place to clearly define the care. The power of attorney is given to a legally designated person, frequently a family member who has the legal decision-making power for Mom and Dad when they are not competent to make their own decisions. Family members and care providers are in agreement that Mom or Dad should not leave the care community without an escort. This decision is made to ensure their safety. Unfortunately, Dad is usually the only person not in agreement with this decision, and he may exercise his perceived freedom and attempt to leave unescorted.

Initially, to divert Dad's attempts at elopement, it is important to *not* tell him that the present care environment is for the long term. For Dad, the idea of such a permanent arrangement may be difficult to comprehend and accept. When Dad hears of not going to his version of "home," he may immediately block compliance with the care environment. He may begin behaviors that may be more difficult to manage, going beyond verbal or casual attempts to leave. Dad was always in control of his destiny during his adult life, and he may believe he has successfully managed the lives of his family, including the adult children.

He may not be compliant with limits placed upon him, such as not being allowed to leave the community. However, the adult children are now in charge of deciding where Dad lives and who will take care of him. It may be difficult for Dad to accept that he has lost his decision-making power and control of his domain and future. Previously, he was familiar with overseeing his children's safety and future, but now his adult children have the responsibility for *his* future.

Even slight changes for Dad may be stressful for him. Therefore, major changes, such as a change of home, may have a great impact. Psychologists note that the biggest stresses for people are high-impact changes, including:

» a change in job,

» change of the home location,

» unwanted change of support systems,

» death of a family member,

» divorce.

The collective effect of these life-changing, stressful events may seem to be happening to Dad as he enters a new environment for his living and care.

Less Change Is Best!

Another strategy may minimize the stress of change in Mom or Dad's environment and possibly decrease elopement. The new living arrangement may be modified to make it seem similar to Mom or Dad's home. This strategy may involve minimal effort, such as bringing Mom's personal items and trinkets to her new place of care. In this way, the new environment is staged similar to her memory of home. This may include using the same mattress, bedroom furniture, and personal items, such as the hair brush from her prior home setting. It may be helpful to place personal items in the same drawers or on the same place on a dresser.

The adult child might think back to the first experience of changing locations, such as leaving home to go to college. It might have been comforting and familiar to bring the bedroom decorations from home and transplant them into the college dormitory.

Another key point to helping one or both parents change their place of "home" is to rely on the experts to guide the process. The personnel at the new place of care may have good advice. Professional staff may have previous experiences that can be very helpful, regardless of whether the place is a group home, independent-living community, or assisted living community. The adult children may want to do whatever seems easier or quicker, with a minimal amount of work. However, changing a parent's environment is a new experience, and it is wise to acknowledge that the experts may know how to best facilitate this transition.

Caregivers will help coordinate the change of the home setting for elderly parents. They may meet with family members and listen to observations about Mom or Dad. It is important to understand the parent, the relationship he or she has with family members, and any fears present. The smoothest transitions often occur when the family members acknowledge and heed the advice of the experienced staff.

Passing the Baton

A successful transition can occur when the family trusts the staff with the process of changing home for Mom or Dad. Pat was a lady I had known for many years because she had been in the business of assisted living and had chosen to place her father in the assisted living community that I directed. Pat was familiar with all aspects of assisted living operations, but I was concerned that she would be reluctant to delegate responsibility for her father's care to our staff. She was not prepared for some of the behavioral patterns from her father that many people experience when their parent enters a new care environment.

Bill, Pat's father, did not want to leave his home. He was a person of habit, and his home was all he knew. Martha, Bill's wife, was feeling much stress because of his loss of memory and function. Martha was mentally in good health and had no symptoms of dementia. However, Bill's refusal to have any outside help with his care was taking a toll on Martha's health. She felt that she could not continue to make health-care decisions for Bill or care for him at home any longer.

Martha decided to live at their long-term home separately and alone because she needed rest from years of caring for Bill. As a result, Bill was feeling abandoned by Martha. Bill had thought that everything was just fine at home, and he felt it was her responsibility to care for him. After all, Martha had agreed to care for Bill when she took marriage vows fifty-five years earlier.

Martha and Pat agreed that it was time to move Bill to an assisted living home. They needed reassurance that this was the right thing to do, because Bill was so resistant to the idea. As Bill's nurse, I suggested that it would be best that Bill move to the assisted living community; otherwise, Martha's physical and emotional health would decline because of the stress of taking care of Bill at home. By reinforcing what they already knew, Martha and Pat felt much relief.

The family did exactly what was best because they heeded staff guidance from the start. As a result, a potential struggle concerning the transition was averted. Although they saw themselves as experts, they understood that they were in the family role and needed to step back from hands-on care and place their trust for Dad's care with the staff. They respected the experts in the assisted living community because these experts had years of experience and success. Pat relied on staff expertise to guide her and her mother regarding how to tell Bill about his forthcoming move.

After the move, the family trusted the staff with what to say and do when Bill wanted to go home or missed his wife. Within six weeks, he had made the adjustment to his new home. This smooth transition was facilitated because his family relied on guidance from the staff. The family realized that they were too close to the situation to be objective. A potentially catastrophic experience became a good move for Bill, minimizing the stress on all family members, including Bill.

CHAPTER 5

Behavior and Symptom Management for Memory Loss

I. Embracing Elopement

When a Workday Never Ends

Elopement is the attempt of dementia residents to leave the place of care without authorization. Dick, eighty-four, was a hard-working professor his entire working life, but he had not worked for at least fifteen years. In his state of mind with progressed dementia, he still believed he had his job and felt the work environment at the office could not exist without him. Every day, he needed assistance with every aspect of care. However, he could do one thing on his own: he would take his briefcase, pack it with papers, and head for the door to go to work. Despite everything we said or did to convince him otherwise, nothing deterred Dick from this behavior pattern.

In his mind, people at work needed him. *He knew this place was not work,* and he intended to do everything in his power to get there. We tried everything to prevent elopement with this resident. We engaged him in activities similar to his work. We connected him with other male residents that enjoyed work as he did. We placed signs on his apartment door with his name and work address to give the appearance that this was his office. And we arranged for the physicians to order medications to minimize his agitation and delusions.

An electronic security alarm bracelet (WanderGuard®, Stanley Healthcare Solutions) was placed on Dick's wrist. It triggered a front door alarm, alerting staff when he attempted to exit the community. Dick knew the bracelet was not part of his normal work attire, and he was a master at removing it. When the alarm bracelet was placed in his work briefcase, he discovered it, removed it, and headed out the front door without setting off the alarm "to go to work."

After brief discussion, he usually became very cooperative and gladly reentered the community. However, the last straw was when an alarm sounded after a screen to his apartment window had been disengaged. Staff entered the apartment minutes later to find the window open, the screen off, and Dick gone. Although this situation occurred years ago, I am still amazed that Dick could have climbed out the window. He had Parkinson's disease and was very rigid and slow in his movements. In his escape, he had climbed out the window and jumped five feet to the ground below.

Family and police were notified of Dick's escape from our community, and eventually he was returned by the police. I examined him from head to toe, and he had neither scratch nor bruise despite his escapade. Unfortunately, this event proved that Dick could not safely stay at our community. His family and I met and decided to transfer him to another care community that had a higher level of security. Dick's new home had a front door that was difficult to find, an elevator that added complexity to any escape attempts, and windows that were secured.

This approach was successful. In his new environment, Dick never could find the front door. He walked the halls with his briefcase much of the day and never eloped again.

The Great Escape

Elopement by residents with dementia typically occurs during the first six to eight weeks in a new care environment, when the resident is becoming acquainted with the new setting. There are other instances when the elopement behavior may continue after this initial "getting acquainted" period, and these will be discussed later in this chapter. In contrast, some residents who are more alert and aware may experience a "honeymoon period" during which they initially seem to like the community and show no indication of leaving, but then they change their mind and decide that it is time to head home.

Regardless of when elopement occurs, elopement behavior is very difficult for staff to manage, and it can cause the family to wonder whether they made the right decision to have Dad in the alternative living environment. Guilt and helplessness may overcome family members during this time because Dad relentlessly says and shows that he wants to go home.

Why does Dad want to elope? People have varied history or experiences that may affect their perception or mindset about their present and desired locations. Dad may have a story or perception of what is real in his mind, and this will determine his actions. Dad may feel that he must be doing something purposeful, as in his past, and may want to go home to continue with this purpose. This thought process in Dad's mind may trigger his desire for elopement.

The key approach to prevent Dad from trying to elope involves two steps. First, we try to understand the purpose that Dad feels he must accomplish by leaving the community. Then we take measures to redirect him from this purpose. Each person has his or her own reason for wanting to leave and continue some life purpose, remembered as important. This purpose may not have been part of Dad's routine for many years, but his memory convinces him that this purpose is current.

In some cases, elopement can be solved by creating a similar environment or purpose to replace where Dad wants to go. If he is heading out to work (even though he has not worked in twenty-five years), he can be diverted with tasks that simulate his past work environment. With this solution, Dad will have his purpose fulfilled and possibly lose the desire to continue this purpose elsewhere.

Mom may have the desire to leave to go see her parents, long ago deceased, to fulfill a missed feeling of being needed or loved. Redirecting her to new friends in the community who will care about her, and whom she can care about, may replace this need and prevent her from eloping. In other instances, the solution may be to connect with staff members who care for Mom, and she may see them as familiar and loving as family.

Creativity is the key, especially for people with dementia who do not remember events from minute to minute. In my experience caring for the elderly, placing a simple sign such as "wet paint" on the exit door may deter a resident from touching the exit door to leave. The goal is to keep Mom safe in the care community because she cannot exist alone safely in the outside world.

Return to 404 Hummer Street

Tim was referred to us from another assisted living community that had no systems to provide even moderate redirection from elopement. At the time, he was not severely at risk for elopement, and I felt we could provide a safe environment for him. After evaluating him as having a mild risk for elopement, our plan was to provide him with redirection from staff, with activities that would give purpose and keep him busy. Our backup plan was the security-bracelet alert system to notify staff when Tim was near an open door or when he opened a door himself.

Tim was charming and alert, but he lived in the past. He was physically healthy and robust for his eighty-six years. He had been a paratrooper in World War II and the Korean War, and he reminisced about his experiences in the air force. Tim sat with other residents and staff for hours, telling stories from his past in World War II, and he graphically described jumping from airplanes to escape danger or near-death experiences from his time in combat. He was a detailed and entertaining storyteller, and he could even remember the eye color of his commanding officer from years past. However, his short-term memory was nonexistent. Tim's wife had recently died, but he did not remember that this happened or that he moved to the Seattle area months ago to be near his son.

In his mind, Tim's present world consisted of living, as he did most of his life, in a New Jersey home with his wife and kids. His entire day was spent trying to get back to his home in New Jersey, located at 404 Hummer Street. This address had been his family home where he and his siblings had grown up and where he had raised his family, but since then, other people had owned this home for many years. When Tim was in our community, he wrote letters to his brother at this address. I saved these letters for his son when he visited. The letters were very telling of Tim's thought process of living in the past, as illustrated by this letter that I saved:

Dear Hank,

I'm still in the army. They have me living at the address on the envelope. It's not a hospital. It's just a place they send people like me, a rest home. I'm feeling good. I hope you are still at 404 Hummer Street.

If you are still at 404, drop me a line. It's the same address on the envelope. Write a letter. Hope to hear from you soon. I have been sick some time.

Your loving brother,

Tim

Just sending $10.00 for luck

At first, during the day, Tim engaged in conversations and activities but never attempted to leave the community. He seemed happy and made friends easily. During the evenings, for the first several weeks, Tim played bingo, went on outings, and participated in social activities. At times, he became the entertainment himself. With his animated storytelling of wartime adventures and his outgoing personality, he entertained large groups of other residents. But eventually, Tim became more and more confused, and as evenings progressed, he became a different person.

Health-care providers call behavior differences between days and evenings "sundowning." The sundown syndrome includes a decline in memory and an increase in unwanted behavior and mood changes that appear in the afternoon or evening. Tim did not exhibit these unwanted behaviors in the early part of the day, but he did so in the evening, and this necessitated a completely different plan of care.

Causes of the sundown syndrome can be varied and difficult to establish. Some causes include:

»   fatigue,

»   changes in sunlight,

»   sensitivity to the change in routine for the evening,

»   adverse effects from medications.

At first, Tim's symptoms of "sundowning" included his repeating that it was time to go to his home at 404 Hummer Street in New Jersey. As his symptoms progressed, Tim called taxis, believing he was a short drive from the New Jersey address, which was his destination. Taxis arrived and left after the situation was understood. Staff placed an address plate on the door of Tim's apartment with the address "404 Hummer Street." For a week or more, this seemed to satisfy Tim, and he looked for that address on his apartment door to cue him to enter.

One evening after dark, Tim was determined to go home, and he walked out the front door. The staff was unsuccessful in redirecting Tim from the door, and they followed him. They attempted to convince him to come back to the assisted living home or to call his family or a cab. It was rush hour, and cars were bumper-to-bumper on the street outside the community. Tim did not pay attention to the cars or traffic lights. He walked across the street with cars screeching to a halt, and he ignored the staff's desperate attempts to redirect him with conversation back to the safety of the community.

The police and family were called to assist, but they had not yet arrived. Tim's delusion was extreme, and he thought he still was in the army and being held captive by two Hispanic male staff. The care staff desperately attempted to get Tim back inside, but he resisted further and started to fight these "enemy soldiers," swinging at them and yelling for help. Bystanders watched as two young men seemed to be having a confrontation with an older Caucasian man.

By the time family and police arrived, Tim was safely inside the community with no memory of the situation at all. Tim's situation did not improve, and he was admitted to the hospital for medical management of his delusions. Eventually, he was placed in a skilled care community where one of the nurses had an amazing, almost identical resemblance to his late wife. She resembled his wife of thirty years ago, with similar appearance, weight, height, and a New Jersey accent—just how Tim remembered her. Tim's elopement attempts stopped at the skilled care community when he connected with this nurse, convinced that she was his wife.

Home Improvements Gone Bad

Chris never tried to elope from our community until the day his carpet was replaced. The strangers in the apartment who were changing the carpet, and the slight difference in the environment, caused him to become confused. The apartment was not the same, and he decided that he would not stay there. Chris sat near the door as he always did, watching people. Eventually, he was ready to go home, but instead of going upstairs to his apartment, he headed out the front door.

A community event had just ended, and many people were coming and going. Chris joined a large group of people heading out the door, and he left undetected. As he had not been considered at risk for elopement, he did not have a security alarm bracelet, and no door alarm sounded to alert the staff. Chris walked to the bus stop a hundred feet away and got on the bus. Chris would have been unable to pay, even if he had money, because he had advanced dementia and did not communicate with strangers.

It was dinnertime before anyone noticed Chris's absence, and he was nowhere in the building. The staff checked every apartment, according to protocol, and then went out in cars combing the streets. Police were called to assist, and he was finally found at a Park and Ride in the next town. The bus driver had alerted somebody for help.

Although Chris returned to the community safely, it was important to recognize what triggered his elopement in order to avoid a repeated incident. In his case, elopement was triggered by a disturbance in Chris's environment that had felt safe and secure until it was "invaded" by strangers who came to replace his carpet. After the strangers entered his apartment, Chris felt unsafe. The additional change in the new carpeting created another unfamiliar feeling that caused him to lose a connection of comfort.

When Nurturing Never Ends

I cared for Rachael, in her late eighties, when she lived in our assisted living community. Throughout her life, her most significant purpose was caring for family, including her husband, children, grandchildren, and great-grandchildren. Eventually, after years of dementia-related care, Rachael died. I went to her memorial service, where many family members and friends reminisced about their memories of Rachael.

As members of the family stood up and recited memorable experiences with Rachael, I realized how different my experience with Rachael had been. I had known Rachael only when she had significant dementia. Rachael rarely had visitors at the assisted living community. Therefore, family members and friends at the service knew her only from previous, active times in motherhood, when she was brave, adventurous, or the life of the party. Each time a member at the memorial service stood up to relate a special memory about Rachael's past, the entire congregation could relate. Yet I recalled Rachael's years with dementia, living in the assisted living community, including her confusion and her constantly wanting to go home to take care of her babies.

At the memorial service, I met Rachael's family members— the people that Rachael had viewed as her babies who needed her care. These were the most meaningful people in her life, so I decided to tell a story about Rachael and my experience with her in assisted living. I had experienced Rachael's passion for caring for her family, a passion that caused her to attempt to elope many times from the assisting-living community to make sure they were safe.

Most people at the service had not visited Rachael during the time of her memory decline or her stay at the assisted living community. Therefore, Rachael's behavior with her dementia was unfamiliar to them. I described how Rachael spoke endlessly of each of her babies, who now were all present at the memorial service, listening to me as adults. I described how Rachael repeatedly wrote letters explaining how she must get home to take care of her babies and was always worried sick that they were not being cared for in her absence. She desperately had written the letters in hope of getting information about their whereabouts. Here is a sample of her many letters (I had stacks of them):

> Dear Sally (her granddaughter),
>
> This is Rachael. I'm trying to find my kids but can't reach anyone. I need some help from someone, so I can take my kids home. This is Rachael and I can't find anyone to help me or take my kids somewhere where I can find them. Do you know where Mom and Dad are? I want to talk to them so they can tell me where they are and help me get them home.
>
> Rachel
> Please give me a call.

Repeatedly, staff had redirected Rachael from going out the door, reinforcing her needless worry about caring for her babies. With Rachael's dementia and absent short-term memory, this strategy lasted only for minutes. She was so determined to go home to take care of her babies, and she participated in nothing, sometimes skipping a meal to wait for them.

As I spoke, the room was filled with stunned faces because none of the people at the service could relate to my version of Rachael's life story. They only experienced Rachael in a more alert and independent condition before her stay at the assisted living community. I looked at their blank faces in the room as they were awaiting the conclusion of my comments about Rachael and the period of her life with which they were unfamiliar. I continued to explain how important all the family members were to her and that caring for them was all she could think about.

I described one desperate attempt to prevent Rachael from eloping, when I reasoned with her as she and I stood by the door. When I asked Rachael her age, she replied that she was in her seventies. I then asked her the age of her babies, and she explained that they were just infants. I replied that I was a nurse and could not understand how she could be in her seventies and have an infant baby at home. Rachael turned to me and explained, "It just happened!"

Needless to say, the elopement attempts continued, because her passion to care for her family remained her sole purpose in life. Rachael soon became ill, was hospitalized, and never recovered. While I finished relating my experience of Rachael's elopement attempts, I could see how happy her relatives felt because she had cared so much for them, even in the times of her memory decline.

Strategies to keep Rachael safe from her persistent elopement were based on convincing her that her babies were in a safe place. It would have been counterproductive to try to convince her that there were no babies to care for in her old age, because this could have caused her to lose her purpose in life.

Going to the Matinee

Dan was fairly alert, in early stages of dementia, when his family came to visit on a Sunday morning. They went for a walk, took him to breakfast, and eventually had to leave. In an effort to leave without Dan becoming upset or wanting to leave with them, the family took him to the activity room with the large television and video library and told him to watch a movie. The family left while Dan was pondering which movie to watch. Dan decided he was going to go to the movies because he understood that his family wanted him to go. Dan headed right out the front door moments after his family exited, and his family was unaware that he had walked out behind them. It appeared to staff members that he was leaving the community with his family.

Dan walked in the opposite direction of his family, down one block to the bus stop, and got on a #230 bus heading to Bellevue, a town ten miles south. Fortunately, he sat next to a man heading to church and chatted long enough for the man to realize that Dan had no business being on the bus. When he arrived at church, the man called our community and reported seeing Dan on the #230 bus. I was immediately phoned and drove straight to Bellevue.

The first bus I saw was #230. I approached the driver when the bus stopped, but the driver said that no such man was on his bus. He radioed another #230 bus driver, who remembered seeing Dan. This bus driver said that Dan was headed to the movie theater when he dropped him off. When I arrived at the movie theater, just blocks away, I saw Dan standing by himself. He was well dressed and walking with his cane. Nobody would have known that Dan was out of place unless they struck up a conversation with him. Dan recognized me and was glad I showed up. He realized he had made a big mistake attempting to go to the movies, and my showing up indicated to him that God was watching.

On his return to the assisted living community, Dan refused to wear the alarm bracelet to alert the staff about an attempt to leave again. He was aware enough to stand by his promise never to leave our community unescorted again, and he never did.

Take Me for a Walk

Sherri was another more alert resident who did not accept having to live in an assisted living community rather than her own home. Her daughter had previously placed her in a care community where Sherri's repeated attempts to leave created an unsafe situation for her. This care community required Sherri to hire a private caregiver to stay with her at all times, around the clock. The private caregiver was paid hourly in addition to the monthly cost of the assisted living residence, and this was a very expensive solution to address the elopement behavior. The family moved Sherri to our community because they were searching for other solutions. Our community had the electronic bracelet alarm system and more activities to keep Sherri busy to provide a somewhat safer situation.

I hoped to address Sherri's elopement by engaging her in various ongoing activities that had been successful with other residents. Sherri's case was difficult, because she did not like to do projects and activities with others. She was a loner who enjoyed taking long walks. Although Sherri verbalized that she wanted to go home, she actually wanted the experience of a long walk outdoors.

Finally, a solution was reached. We hired somebody to walk with Sherri two hours every day. We gave Sherri a schedule that showed when her walking companion would go out with her, so she could be reminded and anticipate the walks. After she knew that she could go for long walks during these times, Sherri never attempted to leave the community alone again.

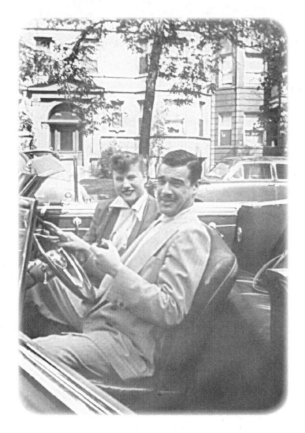

Techniques to Prevent Elopement

Technology is available to help with monitoring and preventing elopement. A Global Positioning System (GPS) device can track people from the community, and a personal wrist alarm band (WanderGuard®, Stanley Healthcare Solutions) can be placed on Mom to notify caregivers of an exit. More than one strategy is usually necessary to resolve an elopement situation; a creative combination of several approaches may include:

»   redirecting Mom's interest,

»   involving her with friends,

»   implementing alarm technology,

»   medical management for unsafe behaviors.

Potentially serious consequences can result if Dad elopes and his absence is unnoticed for some time. If staff do not witness him leaving his care community, he may not be missed until he is absent from a meal, planned activity, or medication time. A young child walking unattended or getting on a bus alone would be alarming to bystanders and would trigger a response, but this is not the case for the elderly adult, who may not appear out of place by himself.

The elderly adult wandering from a care setting may not be noticed because he may appear similar to other elderly people on the street. People who see Dad will be unaware of the level of assistance he needed that morning to don appropriate clothing for that day. Only when strangers speak to Dad will they become aware that Dad should not be alone on the street, and instead, Dad should be receiving needed care, like an innocent lost child in need of direction.

II. Sexual Behaviors with Dementia

People with dementia have sexual desires and behaviors that resurface from the past. Sexual activity is private and occurs behind closed doors, and it may be difficult to understand the sexual desires or behaviors of people with dementia. Adult children may prefer not to consider their eighty-year-old parent with dementia as thinking of sex or having sexual behaviors.

Some people with dementia have sexual desires. They may not connect the desires experienced with the physical actions needed to address these feelings, and they may become agitated. Others may seek out a mate with whom to share sexual relations. Some elderly people may masturbate or have their hands gravitating to their genitals regardless of the social situation. They may manipulate their genitals in a way analogous to an automatic reflex, a behavior sometimes seen in young boys. With Dad's dementia, he is unable to control his undesirable sexual behaviors, and he does not consider the social taboos associated with these actions.

With dementia, Dad may react freely and be uninhibited in his sexual desires. Dad may grab the breasts or buttocks of a woman nearby. He may be inappropriate verbally, blurting out sexual statements as women walk by or in casual conversation. These undesirable and disturbing sexual behaviors are difficult to correct because they are automatic, without forethought. They are usually managed with medication. However, the physicians prescribing medication for Dad must be cautious not to overmedicate him, because adverse reactions may include dizziness and unsteadiness that may cause falls and injuries.

Mom and Dad with dementia may continue to have sexual activity as a private experience. They may be taking their sexual experience from a previous period in their long-term memory. When the long-term memory dictates sexual intercourse behaviors for Mom and Dad with dementia, the sexual activity may be similar to that of couples aged in their twenties rather than their fifties. In the few embarrassing times that I accidentally entered a room with an elderly couple having sexual relations, I have been surprised at the nontraditional sexual activity that I witnessed. Regardless of the time in life that the resident with dementia exhibits this behavior pattern, it is harmless and can be considered healthy.

Beverly's Many Men

Beverly was in her early eighties, experiencing moderate dementia. Her family moved her into the assisted living center because she was unable to take care of her large home. She needed assistance with basic aspects of food preparation and taking her medications. Beverly had a bubbly and outgoing personality throughout her life. She was a cheerleader in high school, and in her adult years she participated in social clubs.

Beverly was a homemaker in her adult years and had two daughters with her husband. She was widowed many years ago but kept herself busy with many girlfriends and an active social life.

In the assisted living community, Beverly continued to be socially active, but primarily with men more than women. She was flirtatious, similar to a teenage girl. Her daughters were shocked because they had not previously seen this behavior as children or adults. Beverly frequently was found sitting on the lap of an elderly companion from the assisted living community, flirting with and caressing him. Later in the day, she might be walking hand-in-hand with a different elderly gentleman, as if they were partners. Beverly's daughters were informed of her recent behaviors, and they decided to consider this as healthy behavior that made their mom happy.

As time progressed, Beverly's dementia deteriorated, and past behavior patterns resurfaced. Her relationships with her male friends in the assisted living center became more intimate. Beverly lured her male companions to her or their apartments and had sexual relations with them. Staff members found her in various sexual acts with one of her several male companions. Beverly was caught having nontraditional sexual intercourse or providing oral sex to her partner. Her daughters had a difficult time accepting this behavior. They considered transferring her to a group home with all female residents, but they ultimately decided to allow her to continue with the behavior that she enjoyed.

Beverly's behavior may have resurfaced from an earlier time in her life before her marriage and traditional family life. Elderly people who have dementia may relive experiences and thoughts from their long-term memory. Therefore, Beverly was probably reliving sexual behaviors from her distant past.

Cathy and Paul: Unconventional

Cathy and Paul were both living at the assisted living community. Both had spouses who were deceased, and they found comfort in their companionship. They both experienced significant memory loss, and they lived in the past, not remembering anything from their short-term memories. Their companionship seemed conservative and innocent. They sat together during meals and entertainment. Occasionally, I saw them walking down the halls hand-in-hand.

One evening, when I was staying late, a staff member told me that Cathy had lost her room key and needed another. I retrieved another key and proceeded to Cathy's apartment to give it to her. The door was closed, but I knew she was there because the staff member had told me that she had let her in. I knocked and then opened the door a couple of inches, noticing that it was dark. I thought Cathy was asleep, so I entered to place the key inside. However, I soon realized that Cathy was not asleep. She was lying down on her bed naked from the waist down, and her bottom was at the edge of the bed with her legs raised up and spread way far apart. Paul was on his knees, fully clothed, with his head between her legs. I realized that he was giving her oral sex. I excused myself and left the room.

The experience was surprising to me in many ways. I was astonished at how agile Cathy appeared, because she did not appear as flexible in the daily exercise sessions in the community. I wondered how this couple knew about this type of sexual activity; perhaps it was from the long-term memories of sexual behavior from their twenties or thirties. I also wondered how long that behavior would continue between them, because they both had progressed dementia with no short-term, minute-to-minute memory.

Tony's Passion for Women

Tony was a very religious Catholic. He had a long-term marriage of sixty-seven years to Peg, and they had seven grown children. Tony was admitted to the assisted living community by his family because they could not manage his behaviors related to his dementia at home.

Tony experienced moderate memory loss and had sexual behaviors that he could not control. When women were walking near Tony, they had an experience similar to that of a young, attractive woman walking by a construction site. He pinched young women on the rear or grabbed their breasts. He whistled at women, told them they were beautiful, and invited them to sit on his lap. Tony could not control his sexual behaviors. His wife and family did not know what to do about this problem.

Tony's physician prescribed various medications that curbed his inappropriate sexual behaviors. Although the medications successfully addressed the problem, they caused sleepiness, unsteadiness, and a fall. However, Tony's family chose to have him continue with the medications rather than contend with other people falling victim to his sexual behaviors.

III The Fairy Tale

There is a fairy-tale-like world in the mind of people with dementia. The mind of dementia intertwines fantasy with reality. With deteriorating nerve cells, pathways of activity in the aging brain do not function normally. As a result, reality and perceptions become twisted.

Some residents with dementia live in a distorted fantasy world, and a false perception may be interpreted as reality. Mom may mistake staff members or other residents as family members or siblings. Mom sees and interacts with these people, and her mind changes their identity to satisfy her desires. She may wake up every morning and see the caregivers, believing they are her sister or mother, especially if the caregiver looks somewhat like that other person. The fantasy is a comforting vision that makes the day a pleasure from the time Mom wakes up until she goes to sleep. The fantasy enables Mom to feel safe with the people or situations that bring her comfort.

For residents with moderate to severe memory decline, there are creative ways to address their dementia-related fantasies. For Mom who continues to embrace the fantasy that she cares for her children or infants, we have an activity station for baby care with a bassinette, highchair, and several life-size baby dolls. For Mom who desires to shop for food and continue to provide items for her home or family, we have a general store setup, with grocery bags, food, and a checkout counter. Items in the store are labeled with prices from the past, familiar to Mom, such as milk for fifty cents or bread for seven cents.

Other activity stations include a desk with a briefcase, an old typewriter for the men who fantasize about going to work, and a mailbox for those who feel they need to get the mail. One of my favorites is the bus stop in the courtyard next to an old lantern, for those residents who need to go home on the bus after work. Dad may go to the activity bus stop at the end of the day and wait for a bus to take him home, as he did in the past. He may forget that he lives at the assisted living community, and he lives the fairy tale that it is time to go home because his workday is done. Mom may wait at the bus stop to go home to her parents and carries the fantasy that they are waiting for her.

The bus does not arrive at the activity bus station in the courtyard, and parents of our eighty-seven-year-old residents do not come to get their child. We redirect Mom and Dad to wait until the next bus arrives and to participate in something else. They reluctantly cooperate, but once engaged in another activity, they quickly forget about their missed transportation.

Sisters Reunited

A fantasy sometimes makes the transition to assisted living easier. Alice came to the community with her family for a visit. It was such an easy transition for her because she immediately saw another resident, Dora, and was convinced that Dora was her long-lost sister. Alice moved in without a complaint or glitch.

Her family was shocked because, until the moment she met her "fantasy sister," she had been adamant about not moving to assisted living. Amazingly, the "new sister," Dora, also had significant dementia and participated in Alice's fantasy. Dora, too, was convinced that Alice was her sister. Alice ate every meal with her "sister," and sometimes they argued like ordinary siblings.

The Perfect Companion

Sally was another resident who had a comforting fantasy that made for a smooth transition to the assisted living community. She was receiving less than adequate care at a very upscale assisted living center in an adjacent town. Sally's family members proceeded with the move to our community, even though they worried that she would miss all her friends in the previous center. Sally never complained or showed behavioral signs of struggling with the transition to our community.

When I went to see how she was doing, I found her sitting at an activity with many residents, holding hands with a new friend, Bill. I asked Sally who this person was next to her, and her eyes lit up and twinkled as she said, "This is my husband." She was so happy to be reunited with her husband that she glowed. I asked Bill if he was okay with this, and he simply shrugged his shoulders and smiled. Fortunately, he was happy to be in a new fantasy of being married.

Awaiting the Queen

Mom's ability to enjoy reliving her memories from past years may help her feel wonderful, happy, and purposeful in the present. Robbeh was Persian and lived much of her life as the wife of a diplomat. Her days had been filled with planning events and entertaining queens and other government officials. She had been groomed for this royal lifestyle and had impeccable social graces, playing the role of the hostess with the proper response to every social interaction. She possessed the art of conversation, and she knew how to ask kind questions with a genuine smile.

After Robbeh developed dementia, she moved to an assisted living community in America, close to her son. The assisted living community was palatial, with formal dining and a grand staircase in the entry. Robbeh lived the fairy tale as if she were living in a palace. Every day, she went to the concierge and asked if the queen would be arriving for lunch. The days were exciting as she primed the staff to await the queen. Many days, she dressed up for lunch or straightened up her apartment or the lobby, in anticipation of the queen's arrival. This was a safe world for Robbeh and a great experience for the staff.

Going to the Mall

Conflict occurred with one resident when her friend did not join in and believe her fantasy. Carol and Winfred were best friends in the assisted living center where they resided, and there was rarely any tension between them. They ate together at meals, always saving the next seat at the table for each other. At an activity, if one was missing, the other would be worried sick until her best friend showed up.

However, this day was different. Carol and Winfred were arguing. Carol was vividly describing a mall, located in the basement of their assisted living center, but Winfred did not believe her. In fact, there was no basement level at the assisted living community. Winfred knew this and persisted in correcting Carol. Carol felt that Winfred was accusing her of telling a lie. Carol, in her fairy-tale world, had been to the mall in the basement many times, and in her mind, this was the true reality.

Carol recalled every store to Winfred in detail, and she told her how she had just shopped there the other day with her son. Carol explained that at the basement level, there were shoe stores with a nice man, great bargains on clothing, and many other shops. This was Carol's comforting fairy-tale world that she could not leave, despite Winfred's efforts to correct her. Carol became increasingly upset with her best friend, and for a time, it was best to separate the two friends.

As a distraction for Carol, the staff invited her to join our staff meeting. Carol joined the meeting and continued to verbalize her distress that Winfred did not believe her, and she asked the staff whether they knew of the mall. Without hesitation, all staff members raised their hands, confirming the existence of the mall in Carol's fantasy world of dementia.

At that moment, Carol felt safe with her fantasy world validated. Carol was happy and calm when she received this confirmation of her perception of reality. By the following week, Carol had forgotten about the mall, and she and Winfred were, once again, together in harmony.

Embracing the Fairy Tale: Live the fantasy with them!

When confronted with the fairy tale, families inquire about how to best handle Dad's fantasy version of the world. When they try to correct Dad, an argument starts. When they tell Dad that he does not need to go to work and has been retired for twenty-five years, he gets depressed. It is never good to bring Dad out of the fairy-tale world, because he believes it to be true. By correcting Dad and bringing him back to reality, children may trigger feelings of sadness or anger, and it may be very difficult to contend with the behaviors resulting from reality correction. It is easier and safer to allow Dad to continue living the fantasy of the fairy tale, because the world of the fairy tale is pleasant and safe (unless it is the nightmare, discussed below).

Dad may view reality as unpleasant, and this may cause him to feel frustrated, anxious, or angry. For this reason, I always recommend that families and staff enter the world of Dad's dementia fairy tale and not try to bring Dad to our reality. Dad's fairy-tale thoughts are analogous to a distressed child's ability to pretend and seek pleasure or safety. Dad with dementia will seek a "fight or flight" response by entering the fairy-tale world for comfort. Although our minds are more mature and worldly as adults than when we were children, we continue to seek the same comfort response when distressed.

Dad experiences distress from the lack of familiarity with his environment, and he sees nothing as he once remembered it. He tries to make sense of the unfamiliar present situation by connecting with familiar memories from the past. Some of these past memories may be relived in twisted versions that differ from the past reality. He transforms what he sees in his present surrounding environment to fit into a version he remembers from a past situation. This becomes Dad's new version of the reality that he embraces. It is difficult to convince Dad that he has created a false reality. Problems occur when families or staff members are not supportive of Dad's perceived reality.

Reunited with Sister

William, a new resident at the assisted living center, had moderate memory loss. He saw nothing familiar to him at the assisted living community, and he was scared and lost. However, all his fear evaporated several days after arrival when he laid eyes on Peg, another resident living at the community. William was convinced that Peg was his younger sister, Clare. In his mind, he was now safe in the presence of his sister. From that day, William repeatedly searched the assisted living center for Peg. When he found her, he referred to her as Clare and badgered her in the way he had harassed his sister, Clare, as a young child.

Peg also had dementia, but she was aware enough to know that she did not want to be Clare. When Peg told William that she was not Clare, William argued with her and became agitated. It became necessary to keep William separated from Peg, and William was moved to a different section of the assisted living community.

IV. The Nightmare

Although some elderly people with dementia live in a fantastic fairy-tale world, others live in a darker version of reality similar to a nightmare. Those who live the nightmare remember dangers from their past, and they believe that these bad experiences are occurring in the present. These negative memories create a "doom and gloom" reality, keeping the resident in constant fear of harm or danger.

A manifestation of the nightmare may occur when Dad has forgotten all that is familiar to him, and he does not recognize people or routines. In this situation, he lives in fear of the unfamiliar, with no stability in his life. When this happens in early stages of dementia, Dad may simply withdraw and remain quiet. He may choose to be alone and avoid addressing the unpleasant fears of the unfamiliar. In late stages of dementia, Dad may become nonverbal, and he may react by acting or lashing out because this is his only available defense against the dangers that he perceives.

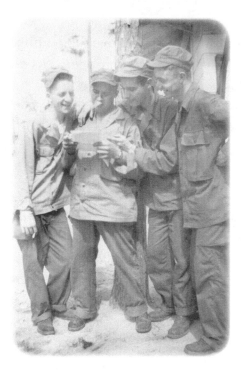

The Prisoner of War

Nan and her daughter Debbie visited our community in desperation. Joe, Nan's husband, was in his eighties and was living in an adult family home. He had become unmanageable because of violent and belligerent behavior, shouting and trying to hit the care staff and Nan. Joe had been asked to leave the adult family home. Nan needed to find a place quickly for Joe. He had no history of violent behavior in their forty years of marriage, but recently this had become a regular occurrence.

After meeting with Nan and Debbie, we decided to have Joe attempt a stay in the assisted living community. A plan of care was needed to address his present behavioral issues. Joe was living a nightmare reality of the experience he had many years ago as a prisoner of war during World War II. He associated the confines and rules of the group home as similar to the prisoner experience from his past.

To break Joe from living in this nightmare after he moved to the assisted living center, several key elements were involved in his care plan:

1. **Familiar items from his home were brought in** to help Joe associate his new apartment with his past home, not a prison.

2. **Regular routines** were arranged with the same staff for daily care to help build trust and friendship with his care providers.

3. **A quiet environment** was created to promote calmness.

After Joe came to the community, he had an adjustment period of several weeks. As he became more familiar with his environment and routine, his episodes of belligerence gradually decreased. Eventually, his violent behaviors and fears subsided, and he felt secure, knowing he was not in prison anymore.

Money Matters

Another version of the nightmare reality may occur for Mom experiencing dementia. She loses her ability to be responsible for basic survival skills, such as managing her finances. Frequently, adult children assume this responsibility for her, and she lives with the daily nightmare of envisioning that her children may be unable to manage her money and may squander it.

Mom may feel that her own child is the enemy, stealing her hard-earned life savings. Mom loses the sense of trust in her children or others. The paranoid thoughts may make no sense, analogous to fairy-tale-type delusions with dementia, and this nightmare version of reality is very unpleasant for Mom and her children.

Jackie had three children who managed her bank accounts and all financial matters. Jackie became suspicious that her children were conspiring to use her money recklessly. Her relationships became strained with the children, who were managing the funds in good faith. On every visit, Jackie and the adult children had arguments about the financial details. The children became exhausted with the unpleasant visits, and the visits became less frequent. As a result, Jackie's nightmare grew stronger. She envisioned her adult children too busy to come visit because they were spending more of her money on their vacations. The three children decided to explore ways to draw Mom from her nightmare of her children squandering her hard-earned money.

They decided to bring up all aspects of Mom's expenses before she had a chance to approach the matter. This upfront approach gave her the feeling that the children were not hiding anything. After many months and endless conversations to reinforce where the money went, one of the adult children found a way for Mom to be less fearful in her nightmare of mistrust. She started to involve Mom in her monthly account reconciliations by reviewing printouts of her account activity with her.

Whom Do I Trust?

Some people with dementia have nightmares that are paranoid-type delusions of other people misspending their money. At other times, the nightmare may include memories of dangers from distant past experiences that resurface in Mom's mind. These past dangers have a strong impact on memory and may resurface because they are stored in the stronger memory pathways in the mind.

The mind with dementia initially loses short-term memories, but persistent memories may include significant or impactful memories, such as those involving survival, hurt, or danger. These memories sometimes resurface from early childhood. The delusions created with negative childhood memories add to the nightmarish world of danger in Mom or Dad's mind.

If the dangerous memory is from a violent episode, Dad may think that all people are out to harm him and that it is unsafe to be with anybody. This fear of trusting others regarding physical safety is common with elderly people who had abusive childhoods. Their minds create a reality of fear and a lack of trust in others, where everyone is a monster and an enemy.

This is a lonely situation and very scary for Mom or Dad. The "fight and flight" instincts surface from the will to survive, and sometimes Mom and Dad become violent to protect themselves. When care staff attempt to assist in bathing or dressing, Mom or Dad may perceive them to be threatening and may lash out in defense. The delusions are difficult to manage because, similar to fairy-tale delusions, redirection to the real world is not believed, remembered, or understood. In Mom or Dad's nightmare, adult children or care staff members are viewed as dangerous people who can be harmful.

Managing the nightmare reality is very difficult. All attempts are made to help Mom feel loved and safe, and it takes time to gain her trust. Caregivers must listen and provide a gentle, consistent approach when delivering care. The gentle approach includes permitting Mom to decide the next step in her care without being rushed. This consistent approach will gain her trust in the care staff by giving her comfort and helping her feel safe. It is most important to help Mom feel safe, and this priority will dictate how her care should be given.

The last resort for ongoing violent behavior is the use of medications to curtail these behaviors in response to the nightmare reality. Psychotropic medications can help bring Mom to the "edge" of a calm, safe world, enabling her to be more open to reason. She can be led through conversations that build trust in the real world outside the nightmare. Medications may have a side effect of mild sedation, but this effect is not the primary desired intention and may serve no benefit. Doses of psychotropic medications are adjusted carefully to prevent oversedation.

Sundown syndrome, mentioned earlier, is one of the behavior

patterns that may surface during the afternoon or evening hours. Sundown syndrome can aggravate Dad's unwanted behavior while he is living his nightmare fantasy because "sundowning" may change his perceptions of reality. Staff and family must be aware that residents with perfect behavior in the morning or midday may enter the nightmare world of their reality late in the day.

"They're Coming to Get Me"

Sam's nightmare world developed in his beginning stages of dementia. He realized that he was progressively losing his memory. He was divorced and alone, but he knew what he had to do. He arranged a private and confidential meeting with his ex-wife, Sara. Although they had been divorced for many years, they remained friendly and cared for each other. Neither Sam nor Sara had remarried, and they continued to support each other as good friends when needed.

Sam confided in Sara information that she found unbelievable. He said that he had worked in the Central Intelligence Agency (CIA) for his entire working career, never as the salesman he had always claimed. In fact, it was true that Sam had worked for the CIA, and this was not a delusion. Sam explained that it was important that she know about this because he had a government pension plan that had to be managed. He explained that he was losing his memory and decided to entrust his estate to her to manage in his decline. This was the start of a new chapter of their relationship. Sara would be compensated financially for her oversight of his care. He did not have anyone else that he could trust, and Sara agreed.

Sam developed progressive dementia-induced delusions. In his delusional state, he reentered the world of secret intelligence. Initially, the delusions were minimal and unnoticed by others. He became skeptical about trusting people and cautious about speaking or sitting with people at meals. As his condition declined, Sam became increasingly obsessive about how things were arranged in his room. Everything had an exact spot, and housekeeping workers were not allowed to enter his apartment because they might disturb something and place it out of order.

Sam's dementia and paranoid delusions progressively became worse. Everybody had become a spy, and everyone was the enemy. At all times, the blinds and shades in his apartment were drawn, and the lights were off. Unless necessary, he allowed nobody to enter his apartment. Then he blockaded the door, and the staff could not enter the apartment. Until his strength declined, he regularly propped a chair against the inside of the door under the knob or moved the dresser against the inside of his door to prevent intruders.

Eventually, Sam's mental and physical condition deteriorated, and he was moved to the higher care area for increased memory loss. He began to physically resist all care, became combative, and did not trust anybody touching him. Behavior management was difficult, and we rotated staff members until we could find one person he trusted to perform his care. Sam's nightmare of living in the CIA did not respond to medication. His delusions did not end until his physical and mental condition further declined and he died.

Reliving Being Bullied

Stuart had a life story that paved the way for his nightmare-type of dementia. During his childhood, Stuart had the role of being the man of the house. His family had emigrated from Russia to America, and his family struggled for a piece of the American dream. Stuart's father had left the family when Stuart was very young. Before leaving the house, his father physically and emotionally abused Stuart and his brothers. Throughout his childhood, Stuart fought with bigger neighborhood kids or schoolmates who teased him. Stuart became fearful of strangers, but he grew to be very tough and constantly defended himself.

Stuart's physical abuse from childhood and his fear of strangers resurfaced in his mind, late in life, with his dementia. Stuart's dementia was complicated because he had both Alzheimer's dementia and difficulties with memory from several strokes in the previous six years.

With stroke-related dementia, a blood clot may block the blood vessels that feed the blood circulation to the brain, and brain cells deteriorate and die. The memory loss pattern from stroke-related dementia differs from that in Alzheimer's disease. Stroke-related memory loss may not be as progressive as that in Alzheimer's disease. With stroke-related dementia, random memories may be lost, either from short-term or long-term memory. With Alzheimer's dementia, short-term memory is lost initially, and long-term memory loss typically occurs later.

Stuart had behaviors and reactions from his stroke-related dementia that were unpredictable, random, and difficult to control. His distorted reality from dementia caused him to make quick assumptions. He misinterpreted the intentions of strangers, causing him to feel threatened as in his childhood. He looked at unfamiliar people and felt that he was being judged. He reacted aggressively to care providers by yelling at them. Stuart was reliving the nightmare of his childhood, fighting off strangers and anybody else who could possibly harm him.

After a string of profanities, Stuart sometimes realized that he was reacting inappropriately, and he would regret his explosive reaction and apologize. Stuart's family understood the situation and moved him to our community from his home, where he had lived with his wife, Ellen. Stuart's children realized that his behavior and emotional outbursts were harming Ellen's health, because she was experiencing high blood pressure and emotional exhaustion.

One night, Stuart got up to use the bathroom, lost his balance, and fell on the linoleum floor. The staff members knew not to move him because he complained of hip and leg pain and could possibly have had a fracture. The staff honored the family request to call them for emergencies before calling the paramedics. The daughter arrived and noticed that Stuart was very upset and reactive to her. She knew he would be more aggressive in his response to the paramedics, who were strangers to Stuart.

The daughter made him as comfortable as possible on the floor and did not move him. She pulled blankets and a pillow next to him and slept beside him on the bathroom floor the remainder of the night. In the early morning, the paramedics were called. Stuart showed his resistance to the strangers by yelling and swinging at them, despite family and staff efforts to calm him. The situation stressed his weak heart, and he had a fatal heart attack on the way to the hospital. Although Stuart had a fall, his death was likely caused from emotions and stress as he relived his nightmare of fighting off harmful strangers from his past.

The nightmare life that Dad may experience with his dementia is frightening for him, and it is devastating for the family members who watch him experience it. Families must endure Dad suffering through unpleasant feelings that they cannot change, leaving the family feeling helpless. The small, rare moments of touching and being close with Dad must be embraced as they arise, even if it requires a night with Dad on the bathroom floor.

V. The Power of Emotions

Dad's reactions to his daily encounters depend on how well he can interpret a situation and control his emotional response. Dementia will sometimes limit Dad's ability to make sense of a situation, possibly causing him to misinterpret it. He may respond emotionally to a situation differently than he would have before he developed dementia. He may lose control and overreact, or he might not react appropriately to a situation.

Dad's past experiences and learned cultural influences

contribute to his perception of acceptable and unacceptable behavior. This may determine how he responds emotionally to a situation. With dementia, he may be unable to control his response. Cultural influences may create "filters" to guide his reactions, based on his awareness of acceptable and unacceptable behavior.

Typical emotional responses may vary in different cultures. At one funeral, I witnessed outcries and yelling about the family's deceased mother. This reaction was different from the experiences of my upbringing, when the same emotions were expected to be restrained quietly with tears. Despite cultural differences, we continually balance emotional reactions with our ability to control them using our learned societal filters. Dementia can alter these interpretations and reactions.

The effects of dementia on Dad's emotions and reactions can be compared to the effects of substance and alcohol abuse. Drugs and alcohol disable "societal filters" that control emotions and reactions. Rational intelligence is disabled, and emotions take a more dominant role, causing a more extreme response. Drunken individuals act inappropriately. Alcohol disables a person's filters, causing inappropriate behavior and loss of emotional control. Dad with dementia may experience a similar loss of emotional control that may be difficult for families to accept.

It can be difficult to keep a balanced and logical reaction to powerful emotions, such as love and hurt. These strong emotions can easily override societal filters and cause irrational behavioral responses, such as the "stupid in love" response or hate crimes. With dementia, Dad's emotional control may be disabled by his inability to remember societal filters. His reasoning capabilities may be limited because he cannot tap into memories to make sense of a situation. His emotional response may be uncontrolled. Simple incidents and events may trigger emotional responses that are out of proportion to the event.

Families often attempt to curb Dad's extreme emotional responses by rationalizing with him. This approach frequently is ineffective, because he quickly forgets all reasoning within minutes or may not be able to make sense of the explanations. It may require more time for Dad's extreme emotional reactions to "get under control" so he can recover and move to another thought.

Managing Emotions

It is very difficult to manage the extreme emotional responses of Dad who has dementia. Several approaches may be helpful, including redirection and diversion. Medical management is a last resort.

Redirection is the process of correcting or channeling attention. Instead of playing the piano in a setting where Dad is distracted and frustrated, he may be redirected by simply turning off the television or closing the blinds. Simple adjustments to a situation can facilitate the activity.

Diversion is a shift from one activity to another. If the piano playing is frustrating and upsetting, Dad may be diverted to a less upsetting activity, such as going for a walk. The best diversion is a subject of importance to him, which is more likely to attract his focus. If the topic is not interesting enough for him, he may continue to focus on the issue that caused the extreme emotional response.

After Dad's attention has been diverted from the upsetting subject or situation, it is important to keep the new thought in focus until the earlier subject has been forgotten. Diverting his attention is a great strategy to control or dampen an escalating emotional response. We can divert Dad's thoughts by going for a walk outside, talking about other family members, or reflecting on pleasant experiences that he may remember from the past. Sometimes his emotional response can be diverted with music or calming photographs. It is easier for staff to use this diversion method when they are aware of his past and familiar with his fond memories. It is helpful to evaluate what strategies for diversion work best for Dad, because this may minimize his need for medications to address his unwanted behaviors.

Diversion and redirection away from unwanted emotional reactions may not always be effective. In more difficult situations, the family or staff may prevent the extreme emotional reaction by identifying and avoiding the triggering memory or event. In some cases, the presence of a family member may trigger the emotional outburst, and that family member must be removed from the visits.

Some extreme emotional reactions may cause dangerous and unsafe situations for Dad or others in his presence. Dad may become violent or destructive, or he may harm himself. These situations must be addressed by health-care professionals prescribing medication to manage these symptoms. Medical management may be intermittent or continuous, depending on the intensity of the emotional reactions. In difficult cases, inpatient hospitalization in a geriatric psychiatric hospital may be required to adjust the medications. Dad can be voluntarily or involuntarily committed to the geriatric hospital until the psychiatric staff and physician determine the best medical regimen to keep him safe.

Marla's Emotional Attachment

Marla was a ninety-year-old resident with dementia who struggled with powerful emotions of love for her parents. She lived in the past and believed that her parents were still alive. Although her parents had passed away many years ago, she wanted to visit them and believed that they were waiting for her at her childhood home in Bellingham, just two hours away. It was impossible to change her perception of reality by explaining that her parents were deceased. In Marla's world with dementia, she believed that her parents were alive.

Occasionally, the staff convinced Marla that she was an aged adult who had deceased parents. At these moments, she relived the grieving experience, as if it were the first time she had learned of her loss. Eventually, she stopped crying and returned to her childhood memories, believing that her parents were still alive. Marla's days frequently were consumed with trying to get transportation to Bellingham to see them. When Marla heard that somebody was from Bellingham, she became very upset and agitated because she wanted to visit her parents. She walked to the nearest door that she believed would lead her outside to a bus stop for transportation to see her parents.

It was very difficult to manage Marla's agitation about wanting to visit her parents. Marla was unable to accept the reality of the true situation because it did not make sense to her. As a diversion strategy, the staff tried to explain to Marla that her parents were away on a trip. This strategy backfired because Marla then worried about their safety. The staff tried to invent explanations about why her parents were not in Bellingham, but this pacified her just briefly. Within a few moments, she forgot the explanations, and resumed her persistent desires to go see them.

Eventually, the staff members who cared for Marla discovered a successful diversion. They became successful at calming Marla by diverting her to thoughts about a telephone call to a different family member. Her strong feelings for another family member were an equivalent emotion that calmed her. When we informed her that her beloved nephew, Scott, would be calling shortly or coming to visit, her emotional behaviors became manageable. She focused on Scott and her excitement about his forthcoming visit or call. Marla was comforted by believing that Scott was coming to visit. She became calm and participated in activities that helped her forget about Scott's visit. This strategy of diverting Marla's focus to another strong emotional attachment was successful at diverting her attempts to leave the community.

Nate's Nagging Wife

Tina and Nate had been married for sixty-four years. They had two boys, Tom and David, and waited another ten years before having their daughter, Tammy. During the years they raised their family, Tina and Nate were civil and courteous to each other, and they had a respectful relationship even when they disagreed. The children never remembered their parents raising their voice in anger at each other. Tina and Nate contained their emotions, even in the most trying times when they were at odds.

Tina and Nate were now in their mideighties and still living at home. However, their relationship was much different from the harmonious and loving partnership that they had enjoyed earlier. Nate had become increasingly forgetful during the past ten years. Tina assumed a new role of guiding him and managing all aspects of his care. She gave him constant, detailed instructions, beginning upon his awakening in the morning. She told him how and when to shave, how to make his bed, what clothes to wear, and what clothing to put on first.

Nate's ability to contain his emotions became disabled by his dementia. He displayed progressively increased anger toward Tina. He disliked the constant string of her instructions from morning to night. At first, he gently disagreed with Tina, but then he began to argue. The arguing evolved to yelling with rage, and eventually to physical confrontations during which Tina was bruised from Nate grabbing or striking her.

Tammy, the daughter, lived close to her parents and witnessed the abuse in her parents' relationship. Her brothers lived out of state and were rarely in contact with the parents. Tammy intervened and moved her father from the family home, where the parents had lived for forty years. She placed her father in the assisted living community to protect her mother from further harm. Tina remained in the family home to live separate from Nate.

At the assisted living community, Nate was kind, loving, and easygoing with everyone. However, when Tina came to visit, she triggered an anger that he could not control, putting her at risk of being harmed. The unfortunate solution, to keep Nate's anger contained and Tina safe, was to keep them apart. Tammy made the tough decision to stop her mother's visits to Nate. Nate continued to live at the assisted living community, and he had no further outbursts of anger.

Larry's Home

Larry and his wife lived out of state from his son Ethan. Larry and his wife visited Ethan several times each year. The visits were usually one to two weeks and were always very pleasant. Larry had a kind and loving relationship with his granddaughter and daughter-in-law. After Larry's wife passed away, he began to develop the early stage of dementia. Ethan recognized that Larry was unsafe living alone because of his memory loss. Therefore, Ethan invited Larry to move to the Seattle area to live with his family.

Larry's early symptoms of dementia included harmless thoughts that the family redirected with conversation or giving him a task. However, when his dementia progressed, Larry believed that Ethan's home was Larry's home and that Ethan and Ethan's family were the visitors. Larry restricted his daughter-in-law from cooking in the house that he now believed was his. He did not want items in the home to be moved around or touched, believing they were his things. He became very angry with his granddaughter. Larry become very emotional and had verbal outbursts, demanding that Ethan and his family stay out of his space. Larry's behavior was triggered by other people being in his perceived home. After the verbal exchanges became belligerent and foul, Ethan moved Larry to the assisted living community.

Larry began to claim that the assisted living community was his own home, believing that all the other staff and residents were visiting. Verbal encounters became physical, and Larry began to physically push others to get them out of his home. Larry's behavior to protect his space and his home became violent, and he grabbed and hit people in his attempts to force them to leave.

Larry was sent to the emergency room because of his out-of-control behavior. He immediately took possession of the emergency room as his new home, and he became violent to the staff because they, too, were unwanted visitors.

In this unfortunate situation, Larry was admitted to a psychiatric hospital and placed on medications to control his behavior. Medical management was the only effective solution that curbed Larry's reaction to others being in his home.

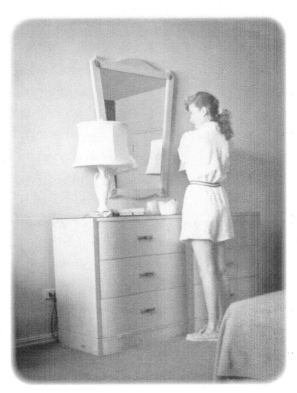

CHAPTER 6

Practical Approaches to Daily Care

Getting Dressed

It is difficult for people with dementia, especially Mom, to dress and change clothes. Mom defined herself throughout her life by her clothing, and she took pride in how she presented herself to the world. This process involved Mom's habits and desires that others are not aware of. With dementia, staff and family take over the process of getting Mom dressed and choosing outfits for her to wear.

Mom's process of dressing was unique to her. She may have habitually donned her shirt over her head before passing her arms through the sleeves, or she may have put on her undergarments completely before other clothing. Although she may have lost the ability to physically dress herself, she is attached to her habitual steps to getting dressed, even though she may not remember them. The staff member assisting Mom with her morning attire may not know her personal preference for getting dressed and will most likely implement what is familiar to the staff member rather than Mom. Mom is aware that something is different, and this may make her upset or uneasy during the process.

Dementia has changed Mom's entire life, and now she grasps for regular and familiar habits. This may include wearing the same outfit every day. Families may complain when they see that Mom is wearing the same shirt again and will not change to a different outfit. When Mom changes the favorite shirt, she will want to go back and change into that familiar clothing item because she has comfort in remembering it as "hers." Even if the clothes are dirty, they are familiar and comfortable to Mom, and there is little you can do to convince her to change.

It is easy to dress a baby or toddler because they are small and recognize you as the authority. Dressing an adult with dementia is much different. Mom is big and accustomed to being in charge, and she often is resistant to another method. The battles and challenges of dressing Mom are much more difficult than dressing a child. Reflecting back to raising my own infants and toddlers, I recall that sometimes they would show great resistance to dressing in the morning for day care. On those days, I could delay the battle of getting dressed until they were more calm and compliant by letting them stay in their pajamas in the car and dressing them at the day care. An adult day care may not be as receptive to Mom showing up in pajamas or dressing in the car.

In the mild and early moderate stages of dementia, Mom knows that there is a sequence to getting dressed, but she may forget what garment goes on first. Women residents often exit their apartments in the mornings with the bra on the outside of the blouse. Mom is aware that a bra is familiar and of some importance, and wearing it in *any* manner may seem logical. Other times, Mom may don several shirts or undergarments because she has lost the ability to monitor or know that one pair is enough.

If Mom has the ability to dress herself but just needs direction with finding a different outfit, we can lay out her clothing on the bed. Sometimes Mom has gone into her dirty laundry basket to find a familiar outfit; if she will not put on another clean outfit, a solution is to lock the closet door with her dirty laundry basket inside.

Grooming

Grooming includes the aspects of care when Mom or Dad is at the sink. They may be shaving, cleaning dentures, brushing teeth, using mouth rinse, or fixing their hair. With memory loss, Mom may remember these details from her long-term memory and continue to embrace them. In other cases, Dad may begin to dislike brushing his teeth and display behaviors that indicate that this is a form of torture.

In people with mild memory loss, grooming in the morning and night may be accomplished by laying items at the sink and giving simple reminders. As moderate memory loss progresses, it may become necessary to provide minute-to-minute and hands-on assistance. With severe memory loss, grooming will require verbal cues and total hands-on care.

Mornings with Anthony

Throughout Anthony's adult years, he performed the same routine at the sink: shaving, brushing his teeth, and gargling with mouthwash. Every morning before work, it was the same series of steps, year after year. When he shaved, he soaped his face (no shaving cream), moved the razor in the same pattern across the right and left sides of his face, and rinsed. Then he brushed his teeth, with a small bead of toothpaste carefully placed in the center of the toothbrush. Finally, he gargled with mouthwash and ran a comb through his sparse head of hair.

Anthony developed moderate memory loss and moved to the higher care section of the assisted living community. Each morning, he stood at the sink and conducted the same routine as in the past, but now he needed help. Although he performed the morning routine in the same order, he could not remember from the previous minute whether or not the task had been completed. He gargled with mouthwash with the exact calculated method of taking in one small mouthful, tilting his head back with a distorted facial expression, and leaning forward to spit in the sink; however, he did this repeatedly until a caregiver would tell him to stop. Although dementia was not affecting his long-term memory about the order of each task, he was not capable of remembering what he had just done in the short term.

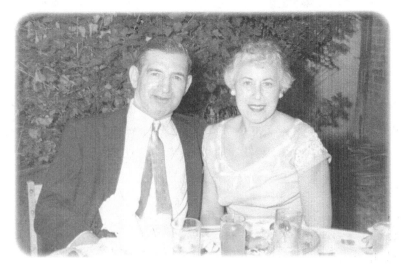

The Dining Experience

The eating experience is the most important part of the day for many elderly people. The meal for Mom or Dad is essential for proper nutrition and provides an opportunity for socializing. Dad may have experienced various restaurants throughout his adult life, or he had meals at home that were geared to his specific taste. The desire for food preferences may not change with the onset of dementia. However, the physical and sensory abilities to enjoy food may be affected by dementia.

Families may be disappointed to see Dad refuse his favorite foods, but these foods do not taste the same to him as they did in the past. Dad does not understand that the food is the same, but *he* has changed. The family wants Dad to continue to enjoy his meals, and they seek an assisted living community where they believe he will enjoy the menu. Families may try a meal for themselves to be certain that Mom or Dad will eat there.

Culinary staff struggle to provide foods that Mom and Dad will enjoy and that will maintain their health and weight. Many challenges exist at home and at the assisted living community when approaching the elderly diet. With diminished senses of taste and smell, a variety of food colors and textures may improve Mom's dining experience.

The taste buds lose the ability to differentiate salty, spicy, and other basic flavors. Some foods may appear familiar, but the taste is perceived differently, causing great disappointment. The ability to taste sweet foods is one of the final senses lost. Many people with dementia crave anything sweet or put sugar on any food items to enjoy them more. The temperature of foods may need to be slightly more pronounced for Mom or Dad to best enjoy them, with hot foods served hotter (but not hot enough to cause injury) and cold foods served colder than in the past.

Promoting Good Nutrition

Nutrition in the elderly is important, and nutritional needs are high. The body may not digest or absorb nutrients as efficiently as in the past. More basic nutritional dishes with fewer calories, starches, or fillers, may be offered, such as pure fish without sauces or gravy. It is helpful to limit refined foods, such as white flour, or foods high in calories. A healthy nutritional program focuses on whole foods, close to their original state, that can be identified from harvest, animal, or fish origin. If you look at a dish and cannot visually identify the food source, it is likely not in its original form, such as a fast-food apple tart compared with an apple slice. It is helpful to read food package labels to check the ingredients and limit undesired and unnecessary additives.

Mom or Dad may need to increase their nutritional intake with shakes and vitamin supplements. Some supplements may cause people to eat less because of gastrointestinal upset or a feeling of fullness. A physician or nutritionist can provide guidance about these supplements.

Other health issues, such as heart, lung, and kidney disease, may further complicate the challenges of menu selection. Patients on blood thinners, such as warfarin, may be on a diet that limits foods containing high levels of vitamin K, such as kale, Swiss chard, or broccoli. It is common for people to be on a diet that limits salt intake, but many foods do not taste as good without salt. In the past, Dad had salt and pepper shakers on the dinner table; now that he is on a no-added-salt diet, he has only the pepper shaker.

The eating experience presents a complex challenge. Therefore, it is important to have a great culinary staff and a team effort from family and health-care professionals. Family may bring in foods from their native country to assist the chef. Physicians may weigh the pros and cons of limiting salt, or the chef may need to provide necessary color changes or "finger foods." Every person has a recipe for success, and individualized dietary programs are common.

Deeper into Dining

People with dementia often try to miss meals because of excuses, such as inconvenience or fatigue. Therefore, in planning meals for Mom with dementia, additional motivational factors may be needed to encourage her to come to meals. Assisted living communities tackle this difficult issue by creating a pleasant, restaurant-like dining experience. They may present a menu with a variety of food items familiar to Mom. Fine linen adorns the tables, and staff members provide good, friendly service. This helps makes the meal enjoyable and convenient and facilitates maintaining high standards of nutrition.

Dad may have lost the ability to feed himself with a fork and knife. He may have better success eating "finger foods." When he needs hands-on assistance to be fed, his dignity can be maintained by moving him to a section with others who have the same needs. If he remains with others more able, he may be embarrassed and not be willing to take the risk of spilling his food. By sitting with others who have the same needs, he is less likely to be judged by his peers, and he may have more success in his attempts to eat independently.

For the aging parent, tactics to improve nutrition can be challenging. Some helpful questions, properly addressed, can assist with nutritional needs, such as:

1. **Exercise:** What physical exercises can Mom or Dad participate in to support brain function by increasing blood and oxygen flow?

2. **Ability to eat:** What obstacles are limiting the ability to eat? Do the dentures fit or need adjustments? Maybe Mom simply forgets to apply denture paste.

3. **Visual abilities:** Can Mom or Dad see the food, or is vision decreased by poor eyesight, outdated prescription glasses, or cataracts? Mom or Dad may not be able to see well enough to eat. Red rims on plates and colored glassware may be helpful.

4. **Food presentation:** Texture variation, appetizing display, and bright food colors can make the meal appear more appetizing.

5. **Medications:** Some medication is better tolerated after meals. Taking medications on an empty stomach can change the taste of the food or cause nausea or indigestion.

6. **Meal environment:** Is the meal environment comfortable or familiar for Mom or Dad? Is it a quiet environment or noisy, busy, and distracting?

7. **Underlying health issues:** Is Mom acting differently? Is an illness or new onset of depression hindering appetite or ability to eat? Medical checkups are important to evaluate the reason for any change in appetite or behavior.

When Did the Recipe Change?

Mary, 102 years old, lived at the assisted living community for seven years. She had mild dementia and was in poor physical health, unable to walk, and confined to a wheelchair. However, the most devastating part of aging for Mary was her inability to enjoy food. Her entire life had been filled with home-cooked meals and fine restaurants, and a top culinary experience was very important to her.

For the first few years in assisted living, Mary was very discriminating with taste, and she was very happy with the food. As her body aged, her culinary experience became less enjoyable because her taste buds became less sensitive and her eyes could not define colors as they previously could. She refused to believe that the unpleasant taste and appearance of the meal occurred from physical changes of her aging body. She blamed the decline of her dining experience on the food preparation by the assisted living chef.

Mary's decline in taste and sight was gradual. Years earlier, Mary noted that she was not able to see color definition and vibrancy as she could previously. When doing crafts and art projects, she had noticed that she could not distinguish between certain colors, or the colors "just seemed different." Mary loved to pass the time by making cards for family members, and color discrimination had been very important to her. She went to the ophthalmologist many times in an attempt to get this corrected; to her disappointment, nothing could be done.

Subsequently, Mary noticed that some routine foods did not have the same taste. At first, she sent the food back, but eventually she adjusted by ordering the same food choices that still tasted good to her. Simple foods, such as egg salad sandwiches, hamburgers, salads, and fruit, seemed the least changed. The texture of these familiar food items allowed Mary to enjoy them, even though she perceived the quality of taste as different.

In reality, nothing had changed with the food. This was the same chef that had prepared Mary's meals during all the years she lived at the community. She was convinced that the chef had changed the manner in which the food was prepared. She regularly complained to her family that the food had changed for the worse. Family members called the assisted living community director, and they insisted on firing the chef because they wanted their mother to be happy with her meals. Nobody could convince Mary or her family that it was actually a decline in Mary's senses of taste and vision that changed her perception of the meals.

Eventually, Mary's family brought in her favorite recipes that they prepared at home. When Mary refused these items, the family realized that Mom had changed, not the food. As a result, the family was more helpful and became part of the team that encouraged Mary to eat despite her objections to taste.

Communication beyond Words

When Mom or Dad has mild dementia, communication becomes more time consuming. Initially, the decline in communication ability may appear when they forget the name of an item or event. Adult children may find that they frequently are finishing a thought or sentence for Mom because she cannot seem to remember. As dementia progresses, communication becomes more challenging, with Dad losing entire thoughts, and random conversations may not make sense.

The adult children know that Mom has an important thought, but she cannot construct the sentence to match the thought. In an attempt to communicate the thought, she may repeatedly focus on a person or item related to the thought, but she cannot put the actual thought to words. This can be extremely frustrating because she may be aware of her inability to communicate. Families are frustrated when they cannot carry out simple tasks because they may not understand what Mom or Dad wants, and they may find themselves in a real-world game of charades or Pictionary.

With extreme dementia, the ability to verbally communicate effectively is diminished or lost completely. The feelings are still present, but their interpretation is up to the caregiver or family member. By learning about Dad's likes and dislikes, family members may better understand what Dad actually wants. If the caregiver is familiar with the person's wants and needs, then the silent world of communication without words can be accomplished using this intimate knowledge and awareness.

Mom's nonverbal communication can be interpreted with tactics similar to those for understanding whether an infant wants a bottle or a nap. The cues are understood by knowing the child and how he behaves when he wants something. Mom, as a nonverbal adult with specific desires, will behave in a specific way to communicate these desires.

Every person uses different nonverbal cues. Therefore, knowledge of past behavioral patterns and desires may facilitate this challenging quest to communicate without words. The subtle changes in facial expressions and the appearance of the eyes may be equivalent to paragraphs of verbal communication. An alternative language unfolds as you speak to Mom in words, and she may respond with a variety of body cues in her new body language. As the adult children become successful in communicating with Mom, they frequently notice that Mom's communication skills may have changed, but she has not changed much in personality. Mom is unable to use words, but her nonverbal facial cues and body language translate into needs and desires.

This alternative method of communication usually changes the way conversations occur. Conversations and negotiations of Mom's desires seem to be superficial interactions and demands instead of the meaningful discussions of the past. The adult children may find that this different quality of interaction is a reflection of the changes in the relationship with their parent.

It is useful to draw an analogy about communicating with an infant. A parent may try to keep the infant awake, hoping that she will go to sleep at the same time as the parent. However, the infant responds based on physical needs rather than logical reasons or negotiated agreements. With moderate and advanced dementia, Mom's body takes control over mental reason, much like an infant's behavior. Mom falls asleep when she feels tired, whether she is sitting in a chair or at the dinner table. She cannot wait until later when she might be more comfortable or when it is time to retire for the day.

Traditional times are irrelevant to the person who has dementia. When Dad is hungry, he wants to eat, regardless of the time of day. Dad may feel that it is time to go for a walk, even though it is the middle of the night. Many spouses of people with dementia describe how they sometimes take their spouse for a car ride in the middle of the night to distract him from going for a walk at this time.

Challenges of Toileting: Incontinence

Urinary or bowel incontinence is the most trying care issue for adult children of a person with dementia. When Mom or Dad becomes unable to control the bladder or bowels, all other physical inabilities and memory issues may seem less important. Incontinence in an adult is a much bigger problem than in a child, because the larger adult has a more unpleasant odor that is more difficult to hide until the urine or stool is cleaned.

Dad may have his own idea of when to change, and not to change, his clothes. He may be resistant to cooperating during the incontinent event because he may feel embarrassed or simply does not see this as a problem. He most likely will not be prepared with the proper equipment needed to manage his incontinent episodes. When he tries to clean up by himself, he may create a bigger mess. On some visits, adult children may find that Dad needs a shower and a complete change of clothing.

The ongoing management of incontinence may cause despair for the adult child because there is no end in sight. The incontinence episodes become worse and more difficult to manage as Mom or Dad declines with age. This is the opposite of potty training for a toddler, because the parent can anticipate a time in the future when incontinence episodes resolve as the toddler matures. For Mom or Dad with dementia, incontinence becomes more difficult to contain and can be the final challenge that prompts a decision to end care at home. This is a turning point for many families, leading them to seek an alternative care situation for Mom or Dad outside the home.

With all the frustration and unpleasantness that families feel about a parent's incontinence, it is important to remember that Mom and Dad also have traumatic feelings about this. They experience embarrassment and humiliation with each incontinence episode, but they may not discuss it or share these feelings. Instead, they may display new behaviors, such as agitation (because of anger) or withdrawal (because of sadness). They may be in denial of their incontinence, as if they want to say, "I am not capable of this, so I did not do this."

It is important to maintain respect and sensitivity to the situation. Mom needs support, not criticism, with these incontinence episodes. Despite the unpleasant circumstances of the incontinence episodes, Mom needs to know that she still is loved. The family can show compassion by sitting with Mom for a few minutes and telling her that they are there for her.

Causes of Incontinence

During mild stages of dementia, incontinence may occur as a result of forgetting which foods cause an upset stomach. By the middle stages of dementia, incontinence may occur because Mom or Dad cannot remember the location of the toilet or cannot organize the tasks to accomplish toileting. In more advanced stages of dementia, the urge to urinate or defecate is not recognized by Mom, and as a result, she may not mention that she needs to use the toilet.

If the urinary incontinence is new, especially if it is associated with new symptoms, such as unsteadiness or increased confusion, Mom or Dad should be seen by a physician. The doctor may diagnose and treat the underlying cause, and the incontinence may resolve. Urinary incontinence may be a result of an adverse effect of new medication. The doctor may adjust the medications, and the incontinence may improve.

Incontinence may be caused by urinary tract infections. These infections are very common in elderly women because the urethra shortens with age and there may be less body fat protecting it. Therefore, bacteria can more easily enter the urethra and cause an infection. Poor hygiene, common with dementia, may exacerbate this problem. Many elderly people are placed on diuretic medications that promote urination and alleviate fluid retention. As Mom urinates more, she may have more moisture at the urethra and the surrounding clothing, and this may create a breeding ground for bacteria.

Preventive measures are best to handle Mom's incontinence. A toileting schedule may be a good solution to prevent recurrent incontinence episodes. Initially, it may be helpful to have her sit on the toilet every two hours until she urinates or has a bowel movement. After she toilets successfully, the family can identify a schedule to toilet her less frequently and better plan outings. It is helpful to bring backup supplies of adult diapers and extra changes of clothing whenever she goes out.

Ambulation:
Getting from Here to There

Dad's daily existence involves him going from one place to another. This may be to get an item, reach a destination, or move around for pleasure. He may have taken this physical capability for granted, and he was accustomed to the physical freedom for completing daily routines. When in good health, Dad went wherever he wanted, on his own schedule, to get breakfast, go to the bathroom, or drive to work.

For Dad with dementia, movement is more difficult, including the simplest movements, such as walking from here to there. He may have poor balance because of weakness, unsteadiness, poor eyesight, or adverse effects of medication. The subtle changes in sidewalk terrain may have become an obstacle course for Dad as he navigates down the street. Getting from here to there has become a challenge for Dad, and the main goal is to avoid a fall and possible injury.

Assistive devices, such as canes, walkers, and wheelchairs, may help mobility during this stage of physical decline. These devices come in many sizes and shapes. It is important to identify the proper assistive device for the appropriate stage of physical decline in order to successfully maintain ambulation and prevent falls. The earliest device for most people is a cane, which is a walking stick that provides a small amount of stability. Canes are useful when Dad has good balance but needs occasional support.

As instability progresses, the walker may provide more stability. For people with declining memory, it is best to introduce walkers early. In later stages of memory loss, it may require much more time, persistence, and effort to learn a new skill, such as the use of a walker. Mom or Dad may be unable to learn how to use the walker because of poor short-term memory.

Mom may frequently get up and walk without the walker

because she forgot that she had it. Therefore, staff or family may need to continually remind her to use the walker. Some walkers have three prongs at the base, and others have pull-down seats, baskets, and brakes. The more complex walkers with seats and brakes are more difficult to master and are appropriate for elderly people without memory challenges. The person using the walker may need to sit and rest occasionally, and walkers with pull-down seats are a great option for this situation.

The more complex walkers have brakes to prevent the walker from wheeling away when Dad is standing up from the seated position. However, these walkers may be hazardous because Dad may forget to apply the brakes, and the walker may quickly disappear as he falls to the floor. Therefore, a simpler walker is better for people with poor memory, and the very basic walker without brakes or a seat is safest.

Electric wheelchairs are useful to provide independence when Mom is physically unable to get around and has no memory loss. However, her slower reaction time with memory loss can cause the wheelchair to hit a wall or another person, or it may fall off a step. The complex wheelchair that previously improved independence can become a danger to others as her memory deteriorates.

The appropriate assistive device for Mom or Dad at the correct stage of memory ability can make the mobility experience safe and help avoid injury.

Managing Falls

Fall prevention programs may minimize potential falls and associated trauma. It can be challenging for people with normal stability to walk with a new pair of shoes, and adult children occasionally stumble. Fall prevention is more difficult in people with impaired strength and balance. Mom may be less aware of her surroundings because of memory loss, and this makes a fall more likely to happen.

Some family members believe that an alternative care center should guarantee that no falls will occur, but this expectation is unrealistic despite an effective fall prevention program. Realistic goals of fall prevention include a low frequency of falls and minimal consequences, allowing Mom and Dad the freedom to get around as safely as possible. If a fall occurs, the alternative care center may ensure that a staff member will be present as soon as possible to assist.

Falls can usually be minimized with common sense measures. Creative measures to provide a safe environment and prevent Mom or Dad's fall may include:

1. **Creating purpose:** If Mom has purpose during the day, she may stay busy and walk less. When Mom is engaged in activities of her preferred interest, she is less likely to wander around aimlessly and fall.

2. **Physical health:** It is important to organize Mom's day to limit overstimulation and avoid fatigue. If she has good rest, nutrition, and personal hygiene, she may avoid physical ailments that could cause illness and associated unsteadiness. Optimal health may help Mom and Dad navigate the physical environment safely and avoid falls.

3. **Mental health:** It is important to avoid anxiety or stress. When calm and comfortable, Mom and Dad may make logical and safer decisions. When stressed or challenged, they may move about impulsively, resulting in disaster.

4. **Safe physical environment:** The environment may be modified with safety measures to accommodate Mom or Dad. It is important to minimize stairs or hills. Minimizing furniture in the apartment or home may decrease the potential for tripping or bumping into something. The bed frame may be removed to decrease the distance from the

bed surface to the floor; this may minimize trauma when Dad rolls off the bed during the night.

5. **Taking control:** Planning activities may include an assessment of the risk for a fall. Moment-to-moment decisions may be hazardous; families may want to avoid conflict by doing what Mom or Dad desires, but they may overlook safety considerations. Therefore, the family can take control, diverting Dad's walk to a time when he is with other people or more steady on his feet.

The extreme measure to prevent falls is to secure Mom with a seatbelt. However, in care settings other than a hospital, it is considered neglect or possible abuse to limit Mom's movement with any type of restraints, including sedative medication or seatbelts. If Mom is secured by a seatbelt in a chair or bed, she is unable to get up when she chooses, and her ability to move freely is restricted. In this situation, she loses her personal right to be physically free to enjoy the basic ability to move about.

Restraining Mom or Dad creates:

»   lack of stimulation,

»   less freedom of movement and exercise,

»   increased frustration.

Physical restraints can be compared to the limited movement of airline passengers on a crowded, long flight, wedged in a middle seat and fastened in their seatbelts. It is difficult to sit in an airplane for a long flight, and it is worse to be restrained in a bed, day after day. Although alternative care situations, such as group homes or assisted living homes, cannot restrain Mom or Dad, the use of restraints is common in hospitals or nursing homes where different regulations dictate care.

When Mom or Dad is likely to fall, care providers attempt to best manage the situation to minimize the frequency and trauma of falls. Mom and Dad need and want to be engaged in movement during the day. Families prefer to have them participate in daily activities with mind-engaging events, and all these activities may create the risk for a fall. When Mom is confused, she may forget that her gait is unstable and unsafe.

Mom wants to continue in physical daily routines but is no longer safe to act independently. She may be unaware that her body has physically changed with increased age. The legs may be weaker than before. Dexterity may be decreased, and coordination and balance may be less stable. These physical changes, coupled with a lack of self-awareness, make walking unsafe and place her at risk for a fall.

Falls are best managed by approaching each person individually, with family involvement. The risk of falling is considered during the planning of participation in quality of life experiences. When a fall occurs, family and staff members hope that safety measures will minimize the severity of injury.

Ilene's Example for Preventing Falls

Ilene was living at the assisted living community for many years. She was a very private person with an old-fashioned and proper manner. Ilene was adamant about being as independent as possible, and she had specific routines in her day. However, she had extensive short-term memory loss. She was frail, thin, and weak. Therefore, she was at high risk for a fall, though she had not previously fallen.

Her plan of care for fall prevention included:

» assistance with dressing;

» assistance with bathing;

» keeping her in the common area where she could more readily participate in activities;

» having staff watch her more;

» using a walker, which helped, and reminding her to use it.

In autumn, Ilene went to bed earlier than previously, because the days were becoming shorter and it was getting dark earlier. As a result, she awoke earlier in the morning after enough rest, when it was still dark outside. She got dressed and made her bed, but she did not turn on the light. In the dark, she tripped on the comforter, which had been lying on the floor next to her bed, and she fell to the floor. The staff came in at the usual time to awaken Ilene and assist her with dressing, which is when they found her on the floor. She was sent to the hospital and was diagnosed with a hip fracture.

When an injury occurs, families become frustrated with Mom or Dad, and they become angry with themselves for not being able to prevent the situation. Unfortunately, falls may occur despite prudent preventive measures. Ilene's family wished they could have prevented the fall by putting a night light in her room to increase visibility or having a care plan in place to have staff attend to her at an earlier hour. These measures possibly could have prevented Ilene's fall, but they were not in place.

In the hospital, Ilene's routine was radically changed. Her privacy was lost because nurses and other hospital staff checked on her frequently, and she seemed sad and depressed. Hospital staff recommended that Ilene recover further at a nursing home, but her family insisted that she should be discharged directly to the assisted living community. The family felt that Ilene would have familiar surroundings and daily routines in the assisted living center, and they hoped that this would improve her depression. However, Ilene was now at higher risk for falling than before her fracture. Therefore, preventive measures were negotiated with Ilene's family to ensure her safety and prevent another disastrous injury. The most likely fall would occur when Ilene was alone.

The plan of care, developed with the family and staff at the assisted living center, focused on fall prevention. The plan included:

» keeping her in the common areas and monitored for safety during awake hours;

» during the night, having her mattress out of the bed frame and inches from the floor to reduce the risk of injury;

» activating a motion detector that would alert staff when she moved, enabling the staff to attend to her sooner.

Ilene's plan of fall prevention worked well, and she had a successful recovery at the assisted living community. She received the necessary care and support from staff and family who were familiar with her needs and were able to care for her. Within a few months, Ilene was walking with her walker, and she resumed her regular activities that she had been able to do before the fall.

CHAPTER 7

Limiting Medications and Improved Health

Strategies to Limit Medications

Mom may have a medication cabinet equivalent to that of a small pharmacy. Doctors and families, eager for the quick fix, frequently use pharmaceutical drugs to try to maintain health. However, these drugs frequently cause dangerous or annoying adverse effects. Improved health can frequently be attained simply by living a healthy lifestyle. Before resorting to medications for Mom or Dad, other methods of health maintenance should be explored, as medications are best used as a last resort.

Various adverse effects of medication include:

» dizziness, which could cause falls and fractures;

» confusion, which can lead to anxiety, getting lost, and limited daily functioning;

» change in appetite, which can lead to poor nutritional status;

» fatigue, which may decrease activity level, resulting in weakness and poor endurance.

Medications frequently have adverse effects that prompt the doctor to prescribe additional medications. Pharmaceutical companies make a fortune from the elderly who are prescribed medications. Mom or Dad may find themselves taking ten to fifteen different medications daily. It is important for the elderly advocate to make sure that Mom and Dad are only on medications that are absolutely necessary.

To succeed with Mom and Dad minimizing the use of medications, behavioral symptoms and other physical problems should be addressed with other creative solutions, not adding another prescription. It may be possible to address Mom or Dad's elevated blood pressure with a dietary change or by modifying the environment to decrease stress. These strategies may limit the need for medication.

Healthy lifestyle strategies that help to limit medications include:

» Emotional support: this can lead to comfort and a positive outlook.

» Healthy diet: better nutrition improves energy, digestion, and immune health.

» Physical activity: exercise promotes strength and blood flow to brain and muscles.

» Stress and anxiety reduction: this may avoid elevated blood pressure and heart problems, and may support living independently.

» Environment: stimulating situations may minimize the risk of developing depression.

Positive Perspective Equals Better Health

Good physical health can be strengthened by having a positive outlook on daily life situations. A positive attitude minimizes stress that can cause wear and tear on all organs of the body and is a powerful tool to reduce anxiety, stress, and dependency on medications. In addition, positive thoughts can actually strengthen the immune system to ward off ailments and overcome or cure disease. Therefore, a positive outlook is a key ingredient to a healthy body. When Mom and Dad experience memory decline, they will be less likely to make sense of a situation. They will be less able to maintain a positive outlook that can promote better health.

Family members must tune into their parent's situation to determine if he or she needs support. They should evaluate whether Mom or Dad has the ability to regain a positive perspective independently or needs assistance to make sense of things. Family members can assist Mom and Dad to regain a positive outlook by supporting them to reenter activities they enjoy. Remembering enjoyable past experiences may include:

- » people who help them feel loved;
- » hobbies that they enjoy;
- » friendships that bring fond memories;
- » reading favorite stories, books, or the daily newspaper;
- » reflecting on favorite places once visited and pleasant times;
- » daily exercise or short walks.

Mom and Dad's ability to maintain a strong positive attitude will promote better physical health and limit medications. With dementia and mental decline, Mom may feel lost in her thoughts and may have increased feelings of stress and anxiety. She may view the daily experiences of life as negative. This negative outlook may cause her to live with less positive energy and can have a negative impact on her health. This may cause Mom to be more vulnerable to illness and to become dependent on medications to maintain her health. Families can attempt to improve inner strength for Mom with positive support.

Healthy Diet Is Natural Medicine

What you eat affects your health. Proper nutrition is another way to maintain health and avoid medications. Eating pure and simple foods with minimal additives can help maintain a healthy body. It is true that "you are what you eat." Healthy foods are pure, simple, and organic with minimal additives. This includes seafood (not farmed), fresh fruits and vegetables, whole grains, and naturally fed meats.

Foods for Healthy Brain Function

The brain is an organ. Some foods support brain function and may delay the processes of aging, possibly preventing dementia, Alzheimer's disease, and depression. Many of these foods contain antioxidants and other substances that work to improve health at the molecular level in the body, including the brain. Some of these foods are:

1. **Berries of all kinds**—blueberries, strawberries, and boysenberries. Strawberries and raspberries are high in vitamin C.
2. **Fish**—Some of the best sources are salmon, tuna, whitefish, herring, sardines, halibut, trout, and cod.
3. **Chocolate**—Dark chocolate is best.
4. **Green tea**—Green tea is a good source of antioxidants.
5. **Grape juice**—Unsweetened juices are best.
6. **Apples**—"An apple a day" promotes general health.

7. **Leafy green vegetables**—These vegetables are a good source of vitamins and minerals, including iron. Iron in the blood increases delivery of oxygen to all cells, including cells in the brain.

8. **Avocados**—Avocados are high in potassium and fiber and may help to lower cholesterol.

9. **Coffee**—Coffee is a source of antioxidants.

10. **Curry spices, such as turmeric**—This contains many antioxidants and has anti-inflammatory effects.

11. **Barley**—Barley may help lower cholesterol.

12. **Olive oil**—Olive oil contains antioxidants, helps reduce the risk of arteriosclerosis and heart attacks, and may improve digestive function.

On visits to Mom's home, it is important to check her cupboards and refrigerator to see what types of foods are available. This will provide an indication of what she and Dad are eating. It may be necessary to coach Mom and Dad on healthier food choices.

With dementia, safety and nutritional concerns may arise, leaving Mom unable to prepare meals by herself. She will require others to assist her, creating a situation where others control her food selection, preparation, and portion sizes. Mom will have choices about the foods that she eats, but she will not have the ability to control her diet independently.

The caregiver who is providing the choices for Mom's diet may focus more on ease of food preparation than nutritional value. It may be necessary to improve Mom's nutrition with vitamins and other nutritional supplements. Vitamins are an important component of a nutritional program for Mom. However, there is a broad range of supplement quality. A supplement that is made to pharmaceutical Good Manufacturing Practices is more likely to have optimal doses of vitamins and minerals and avoid potentially harmful contaminants or additives. A good nutritional supplement is complementary and does not replace proper food intake.

With dementia, Mom's physical health can decline because of poor decisions about the quality of food. Mom may make poor decisions about the best foods, and she may eat whatever she wants. She may not remember when she last ate. With extreme dementia, Mom may experience hunger, but she may not be able to identify what this feeling means and how to resolve it. With progressive memory loss, she also may not be capable of organizing the actions to prepare a meal or feed herself.

Exercise Strategies to Limit Medication

Physical activity may be limited for people with dementia. Mom and Dad may not go on long walks as in the past because their stamina may have diminished or they might get lost. However, there are many modified exercises that can help them maintain good physical health and lift their spirits. This is very important because declining physical health and lack of exercise may lead to poor blood flow and the formation of blood clots.

Family efforts are important to keep Mom and Dad moving and participating in activities to maintain muscle strength and promote blood flow. Simple walks on level terrain may be helpful. Other options include stationary bicycles, yoga classes led by a caregiver, or exercise videos designed for the elderly. Group exercise classes may build strength, balance, and flexibility, and they provide opportunities for social interaction and long-term relationships with fellow classmates.

Hobbies to Limit Medication

Medications can be limited by redirecting and keeping Mom busy with purposeful activities and by managing behavioral issues. Organized programs throughout the day are a great diversion that will keep her busy with constructive activities, decreasing the opportunity to do something on her own that may not be safe. Regular meals with others are an organized, safe activity in which Mom is busy and monitored. Other activities that are engaging, interesting, and purposeful are essential to stimulate her mind. These activities may keep her occupied, helping her to avoid a fall, anxiety, and loneliness.

If Mom is alone too often, she may spiral into a depression that may prompt a prescription for antidepressant medication. Sometimes Mom may not want to join an activity with others and may prefer to be alone. During these times of isolation, she can do meaningful and purposeful independent activities, such as:

» writing letters,

» knitting,

» small projects,

» reading,

» listening to music.

Each person has unique interests. We can help Mom and Dad stay busy and content by getting to know what they enjoy during different times of the day and helping them become engaged in these activities.

Environmental Support to Limit Medication

Many elderly people resort to medications to manage symptoms related to stress, but simplifying their environment may be a better solution. Anxiety may be caused by confusion from living in a large apartment, and this may cause the doctor to prescribe anti-anxiety medications for the symptoms. These medications possibly may be replaced with a comfortable, serene environment and regular routines. The apartment had been familiar and safe for many years; however, with Mom's dementia progressively becoming worse, the apartment is now too big and complicated for her to find her way around. Mom's environment should be set up to help her function easily.

Environments or living arrangements that are unfamiliar or cluttered may cause injuries, such as falls. New injuries can cause a new set of medical problems and added medications, such as pain medications after a fracture. Mom or Dad may have excessive belongings that contribute to stress from the burden of managing, organizing, and cleaning the home. Families can downsize Mom and Dad's apartment or home to a smaller space that is easier to manage, and this may decrease overall stress to the entire family. For people with dementia, an environment with less space can be safer and less stressful. Falls and mishaps can be avoided by clearing clutter.

When placed in a new environment for added care, Mom should bring familiar items so she can feel at home. The familiar functional objects, such as hangers for clothing, may be easier to use and minimize the increased risk of injury that may occur with unfamiliar activities. In addition, people bring photographs of family, familiar trinkets, a musical instrument, or a briefcase that Dad used for forty years. Long-term objects that are familiar and meaningful may be comforting.

Appliances can be an environmental hazard and source of added stress for elderly people. Mom may become confused by the complexity of the controls. The following checklist can help make Mom's life less complicated, minimize stress, and improve safety:

1. Provide simpler appliances. Mom may navigate simple appliances or older, familiar models more easily. Place instructions in large, bullet-point print on all appliances to help Mom use them correctly. Unplug the microwave to avoid overheating liquids and to prevent a fire or injury from a burn; plug it in during your visits, when Mom can be

monitored. Use a coffeepot that switches off automatically in order to avoid the potential hazard of a pot left on.

2. Place a night light. Walking in the darkness is a major cause of falls and fractures. A night light will provide lighting so Mom can find a light switch at night. An alarm clock can be set to awaken her during periods of daylight instead of during the darkness of the night.

3. Provide simpler electronics. Modern television controls may have numerous buttons that may confuse and frustrate Mom. Using an older television with simple controls may be much less stressful for her. Frustration also can be minimized by preprogramming the television controls to Mom's favorite channel and providing simple instruction labels ("on" and "off"). A computer with simple instructions may help navigate her to the programs she enjoys.

Hazel's Polypharmacy

Hazel was a resident who had experienced a decline in health because she had been placed in the wrong environment for her care. The large assisted living community was stressful to her because she did not have a meaningful connection with the activities and people. This situation resulted in an increase in medication with more adverse effects.

Hazel's daughter, Sarah, was her only relative and was responsible for her care. However, Sarah was busy with her work and home duties, and she was exhausted from the additional responsibility of coordinating care for her mother. Sarah wisely placed Hazel in an alternative care environment. However, Hazel's first community was not a good match, and she continued to decline. She was physically and socially active, and she used to walk continuously and randomly, sometimes entering the apartments of other residents or going out the front door. The assisted living community attempted to curtail this wandering behavior by placing Hazel on medications, which caused drowsiness, unsteadiness, and falls with injuries.

Hazel was losing weight because she was drowsy from the new medications and not eating well at meals. She became hungry and ate snacks between meals. The snacks were high in salt content and caused high blood pressure. The doctors placed Hazel on additional medications to decrease her blood pressure, and these medicines caused her to become dizzy and bruise easily.

Hazel came to our smaller assisted living community, and her situation improved. She was happier because she could easily find her way about with fewer distractions. She could always find something to do because she was in a more intimate setting with structured activities that she enjoyed. She was able to interact with others more frequently and find somebody to talk with at all times. In this new setting, Hazel did not have the desire to wander off to other apartments or outside.

As a result, Hazel did not have the wandering behaviors, and she no longer needed medications to keep her calm and safe. The medications were stopped, including the blood pressure medicines, and she was able to stay awake during her meals and eat independently. Therefore, she ate fewer unhealthy snacks between meals, and she experience improved health.

Danny's Diet

Danny was a resident for whom a change of environment resulted in improved health and fewer medications. Several years ago, I had done an assessment for admission to the assisted living community for this gentleman. He was in his mideighties, had memory loss, and was occasionally incontinent of bowel and bladder.

Danny was in his second marriage of twelve years to Carol,

who was much younger. Carol was caring for Danny very poorly because she was physically and emotionally unable to care for him adequately. However, she was compelled to continue because the trustees in charge of Danny's estate had left no financial provisions for her. If Danny was to live separately from her in an assisted living community for proper care, she would have no financial support.

Danny spent much of his day sitting in one chair in a very cramped and crowded home. His lack of activity caused him to become weak and have lower leg swelling. He was not eating properly because Carol gave him the same unhealthy fast-food diet that she preferred. In addition, Carol was unable to assist Danny with proper oral hygiene, and his lack of oral care caused him pain when eating. As a result, he lacked proper nutrition and was eating less, and he was placed on vitamins and nutritional supplements. He became bored and depressed and was placed on medications for depression.

Carol realized that she could not continue to care for Danny and the situation was affecting her health. She was able to arrange with Danny's estate to have him enter an alternative care environment. After he moved to the assisted living community, he was given many food choices that he preferred. The healthier food choices and assistance with his oral care improved his diet and health. He walked more, became stronger, and was much happier being with other people and socializing. Most of his medications were discontinued. The healthy approach to his care in the assisted living community made the medications no longer necessary.

Chapter 8

The Advocate—
Speaking Up for Mom and Dad

I t is common for the elderly to be put aside and lost in the health-care system. Mom, with dementia, can become disoriented in an unfamiliar situation, and she may have delusions or agitation that may be difficult for hospital personnel to manage. Fast-paced hospital health care is not designed for the time-consuming approach necessary to safely care for elderly patients with dementia. It may be necessary to have additional personnel who have special training to manage the elderly patient who needs constant redirection.

Hospitals are intensive environments with time constraints, and patient care must be efficient. Interactions with the patient are usually brief and focused on a specific task. Hospital personnel may treat Mom with sedatives and other medications instead of taking time for redirection and reorientation. General hospitals are not equipped to have confused patients roaming the halls or to provide needed social or engaging activities for the elderly patient with dementia. If Mom is at risk for roaming about and falling, the hospital personnel may use physical restraints, such as side rails on the bed or wrist and body strap restraints.

Mom, as a dependent, needs an advocate to stand by her side in the health-care arena to ensure she gets proper care.

Mom must have an advocate—a family member, friend, or other health-care associate—when she is hospitalized. The advocate must insist on the appropriate tests and make sure Mom is receiving treatment for the correct diagnosis, regardless of cost.

If an advocate is absent, Mom may be unable to communicate her needs or correct any mistaken information. As a result, she may receive unnecessary and excessive tests that may increase the hospital bill. Mom may be left unattended for several hours by hospital staff because she may not know how to use the call button correctly. In addition, Mom may not know how to use the telephone to call family when she desires. She may not be able to nap because the television may be blaring, and she may be unable to turn it off. The advocate is the person who will ensure that the correct steps are taken when Mom cannot serve as a spokesperson for herself and protect her from being lost in the health-care system.

Jan's Support of Mary

Mary, in her nineties, was living alone in her own home. One day, on a regular visit, Mary's daughter, Jan, found Mary very confused. Mary did not recognize Jan as her daughter. Mary had new, dark bruises on her lower back and new complaints of leg pain, suggesting that she had recently fallen. She could not remember where or when she fell, but Jan took her to the emergency room to evaluate the bruises and pain. They waited for several hours until it was finally Mary's turn for an evaluation.

As the doctors and nurses examined Mary, Jan heard Mary answer all the questions *incorrectly*. She even incorrectly stated where she lived. Jan attempted to give the correct answers to the staff, but they continued to write down Mary's distorted version because Mary seemed very believable. The staff members were not convinced that she was confused. Mary explained how she enjoyed independent trips to the grocery store, ate well, was an excellent cook, and enjoyed gardening.

Jan became vocal as an informational advocate and disclosed the accurate version to the staff. Jan told the staff that Mary was living by herself but needed help with shopping and food preparation. Jan explained that Mary had an amazing garden in the past, but she had not had a garden for many years. From Jan's accurate information, it became clear to the staff that Mary was losing her short-term memory but retained her long-term memory.

The doctors initially ordered just a few blood tests because Mary could not communicate her symptoms accurately. Jan advocated on behalf of Mary and clarified the medical history. Jan was familiar with Mary's lifestyle and speculated about the most likely events that caused the fall. Jan insisted that the medical staff should review Mary's medications thoroughly; a complete review of the medications had not been done in several years, and she believed that Mary had been prescribed an excessive amount of medications.

Jan revealed that Mary had a history of urinary tract infections and suggested that another infection could have caused Mary's confusion, leading to the fall. Jan's information about frequent urinary infections prompted the doctor to order a urine culture, which confirmed an infection.

Further tests and radiographs showed that Mary had an old lower back fracture, which could have been disturbed by the fall, causing new leg pain. The emergency room staff suggested that

Mary could be discharged to home with pain control. However, Jan continued in her role as an advocate, and she insisted that Mary be admitted to the hospital to treat the urinary infection with intravenous antibiotics. Jan wanted the doctor to be certain that the infection was being treated completely, without adverse effects.

During Mary's hospitalization, Jan continued her role as an advocate. Mary was more confused because of the hospital environment. Jan noticed that the staff nurses did not go out of their way to check on Mary until she used her call button, but Mary could not remember how to use the call button. In addition, she could not remember the location of the bathroom or how to navigate the television controls. Jan's role as an advocate in the hospital helped Mary become acquainted with this unfamiliar setting because hospital personnel were busy with other duties.

When Jan returned to the hospital the next day, she found her mother sound asleep, unable to be awakened. Mary had been given sedation to prevent her from calling out or climbing out of bed in a confused state. Physical therapists arrived later, but they could not assist Mary with walking because the sedatives were causing her to be delusional and uncooperative. Jan hired a sitter to stay with Mary, enabling the sedatives to be stopped in the hospital.

Mary's urinary infection improved, and the staff began planning for discharge to home. Jan's role as an advocate continued, and she insisted that Mary should have an in-home nurse and physical therapy visits. Jan's role as her mother's advocate helped Mary move through the health-care system and receive the care she needed.

When Staff Stepped Up for Phil

Phil's care staff became his main health-care advocate. He had advanced dementia and was unable to speak. After four years in the assisted living community, his care and patterns of behavior were familiar to the staff. The assisted living staff members could interpret Phil's nonverbal behaviors and reactions and accurately decipher what he wanted. They understood Phil's needs, similar to a mother caring for her infant.

Phil habitually woke up late in the morning, enjoyed the same favorite breakfast each day, and then went about his day with familiar walks in the community. When there was any disruption of his daily routine, such as a different breakfast or a doctor's visit, Phil expressed his displeasure by thrashing his arms and calling out in anger.

During one week, staff members became aware of some subtle changes in Phil. He was urinating less frequently and required fewer trips to the bathroom. The staff encouraged Phil to drink more because the nurse felt that he was becoming dehydrated. He stopped eating his favorite breakfast and became too tired to go for his daily walks.   The family was notified of Phil's changes, and he was taken to his physician for evaluation. On this occasion, Phil's behavior was unusual: he was very compliant to leave the community for his appointment. However, he returned to the assisted living community with no new orders from the physician or explanation for these changes.

After another week, Phil continued to eat and drink less. The staff members at the assisted living community stepped in as Phil's health-care advocate by encouraging the family to take him for another evaluation with his primary physician. His physician gave him a diagnosis of depression and ordered antidepressant medication. The physician felt that Phil was depressed because of a recent room change. Phil's staff members questioned this diagnosis because Phil had changed rooms in the past without having any symptoms of depression.

Nevertheless, the assisted living staff did not give up serving as a health-care advocate. They supported the family and arranged another visit to the doctor. During this third doctor's visit, blood tests and chest radiographs showed that Phil had a respiratory infection that could explain his increased confusion and changed behavior. After a course of antibiotics, Phil became more alert, began to drink and eat as in the past, and returned to his familiar routine at the assisted living community.

The persistence of the care staff was instrumental in Phil's diagnosis and recovery. They served as his health-care advocate and supported his family in bringing him back to the doctor.

The Never-Ending Job of an Advocate

Ted was a long-term resident in the assisted living community who needed the staff to play the important role of advocate for his health care. He was a fragile eighty-four-year-old man with a big personality. Ted frequently walked about the community, socializing and making friends with everyone he met. However, he often became extremely ill when he caught a cold because his body seemed to have weak immunity against infections.

One morning when Ted was getting coffee at the bistro, he turned to offer coffee to another resident and fell straight to the floor, as if he had fainted. The nursing staff quickly arrived to assist him, noting that he was barely breathing. They gently shook him and called his name. Ted was weak, but he opened his eyes and responded to their questions. Paramedics arrived and found that he had a low oxygen level, so they administered oxygen and transported him by ambulance to the hospital. Ted's family was out of town, so the staff, serving as health-care advocates, notified the emergency room about his symptoms. However, Ted returned from the hospital several hours later with no change in orders and no explanation for his fainting episode or low oxygen level.

The assisted living staff members continued their role as health-care advocates. When the family returned the next day, the staff informed them of the situation and recommended that Ted be seen by his primary physician. The family and the primary physician were further informed of Ted's recent cold. At the doctor visit, Ted was diagnosed with pneumonia and treated with antibiotics. His illness was the likely cause of the fainting episode and low oxygen level. After he completed the antibiotics, Ted's social behavior was back to normal, and he had no further episodes of fainting.

In a later incident, Ted fell during the night and sustained a hip fracture. He was admitted to the hospital and had surgery to fix the hip. After a short stay in the hospital, he was discharged to a nursing home. He was unhappy in the nursing home because he was unable to roam the halls and socialize.

As his health-care advocate, the assisted living staff members and his family attempted to have Ted return to the assisted living community. They knew that he would be happier socializing with his familiar friends and enjoying his routines. However, the efforts to get Ted back to the assisted living community were unsuccessful, because the nursing home would not release him until they felt he was ready.

Ted became increasingly depressed in the nursing home and lost his appetite. He refused to eat and became too weak to get out of bed or walk. Despite the best efforts of his staff and family health-care advocates, he eventually died.

The Correct Medicine for Annie

Annie was having her breakfast with her friends at the assisted living community. A staff member noticed that Annie could not lift her coffee cup. Suddenly, Annie leaned back in her chair, with her eyes rolling upward. She appeared to be losing consciousness, and she had irregular breathing. The staff members lowered her to the floor and called 911.

Within minutes, Annie returned to her usual self, as if nothing had happened. Paramedics arrived and transported her to the emergency room for an evaluation. She returned to the community within a few hours, without any new orders. The emergency room doctor had no explanation for the transient change in her condition.

Annie's family was a strong advocate for her health care. They took Annie to several doctors, and tests eventually showed that she was having tiny strokes that had caused the previous episode at breakfast. Medication was ordered to help prevent further episodes. Without the correct diagnosis and medications, additional strokes could have occurred and caused her more harm.

The POLST Form and the Advocate

The Physician Orders for Life-Sustaining Treatment (POLST) is a written health-care directive designed for individuals with progressive chronic illnesses. It is a standardized form in which a patient may specify whether or not they want cardiopulmonary resuscitation (CPR) and other life-sustaining measures to treat emergency care situations. This form is usually held for immediate reference where the patient resides.

The POLST form was designed in Portland, Oregon, in the 1980s by hospitals and insurance companies to limit unwanted medical interventions. It clarifies issues, such as a Do Not Resuscitate (DNR) status, that may not be specified in some living wills. The form supports the desires of the patient and family regarding the life-sustaining measures to be pursued in an emergency situation. It dictates specific health-care measures that are to be delivered by health-care professionals in an emergency or potentially end-of-life situation. The terms for emergency treatment are very specific and clear, and they can be read quickly. The form legally directs any emergency care for residents of assisted living communities, and it may request that no health-care measures be taken, leaving the patient to die in peace.

The POLST form must be signed by a doctor and a person who has power of attorney. Assisted living residents and families may devote many hours contemplating the appropriate health-care measures for a future emergency situation or health-care decline. This process may consume a lot of time, emotion, and funds. The legal documents specify the wishes of the resident and family. Therefore, when the form is signed, it is important for the parties involved to be familiar with all possible situations that could transpire during a medical emergency. This form may dictate critical decisions about life and death, and there may not be enough time to adjust the form when it is required during a health-care crisis.

The POLST form and other legal documents are provided to the assisted living community for reference when needed. In case of an emergency, the paramedics rely on the POLST form because they usually do not have enough time to read lengthy legal documents. The POLST form is written in simple layman's terms and is easily understood. If this form is not on file in times of emergency, all life-saving measures are initiated until the family or other legal documents are located that outline the desired health-care directives for the hospital staff.

In some crisis situations, the paramedics or other medical personnel who interpret the POLST form may not be familiar with Mom and the details that led to the medical emergency. In these cases, the POLST form may inappropriately limit medical treatment. The directives are written very simply, without consideration of specific instances. In these situations, the staff members or family must intervene and serve as the advocate.

Ken's Decision

Ken was a resident of the assisted living community. He had a life-threatening emergency situation, but he was coherent. When the paramedics arrived, the assisted living staff presented them with the POLST form that had been professionally prepared and signed by Ken's son, the designated health-care power of attorney. The POLST form indicated that Ken's status was DNR: do not resuscitate.

However, the paramedics took the best action and served as an advocate for Ken. They asked Ken whether the directions indicated on the POLST form were his current wishes and they should do nothing to save his life. Ken decided that he was not prepared to die at this time and verbally requested that all life-saving measures be implemented. As a result, he received full care, survived the situation, and lived for several more years.

Kurt's Close Call

Kurt was an amazing person who lived in the assisted living community. He had a very sharp mind and enjoyed a very active life. His days were full, working out in the exercise room, trading stocks on the Internet, and socializing with other residents. He and his sons filled out a POLST form and put it on file because he was in his nineties.

Kurt became very ill with diarrhea for twenty-four hours. A week earlier, he had similar symptoms with nausea and vomiting. The staff members knew that he could quickly become dehydrated, and they attempted to give him as much fluid orally as he would take. When the nurse arrived at work early that day, she was informed of Kurt's continued diarrhea and his inability to drink enough fluids to adequately hydrate himself. The nurse immediately assessed his condition. Kurt previously had been a professor and was very articulate, but now he could barely talk or stay awake. He was very weak, lying flat in his bed. The nurse measured his blood pressure, which was very low, confirming that he was dehydrated. He was nauseous and could not drink any more fluids. The only way to give him fluids in his condition was through an intravenous infusion.

Kurt had fear in his eyes, and the nurse knew he was scared. He was well aware of the severity of his situation. The staff called 911 emergency services to assist with Kurt's health-care situation. The nurse explained to Kurt that if he wanted to get well, he must go to the hospital for intravenous fluids because we could not provide the fluids he needed in our assisted living community. Kurt stated that he wanted to have everything done to save his life, and he agreed with our decision to call the paramedics.

The staff followed standard procedure and gave the paramedics the POLST form, medications, and emergency information history. One paramedic was very young, and the nurse assumed that he was new because she had not seen him in any previous emergencies. The paramedics suddenly stepped back from Kurt and stopped any life-preserving actions. They simply reviewed his paperwork and looked at his electrocardiogram. Kurt was barely conscious and was unable to communicate with the paramedics. His blood pressure was very low, creating a life-threatening situation.

The nurse asked the paramedics why they were not starting the intravenous fluids that Kurt needed to survive this crisis. The younger paramedic told the nurse that the POLST form indicated that he should receive no intravenous fluids. She checked the form and saw that he was correct, but this was not what Kurt had indicated to her before the paramedics arrived. The dehydration could easily be corrected, and this was not the type of life-threatening situation for which the POLST form had been prepared.

At this moment, the nurse had to serve as an advocate for Kurt. This was not the chronic decline for which Kurt and his family indicated on his POLST form that no intravenous treatment be given. The nurse argued that they needed to start the intravenous treatment to prevent this reversible condition from taking Kurt's life, but the paramedics did not agree. Therefore, the nurse told the paramedics that the family member who was the power of attorney must be consulted urgently. Valuable time was being wasted, and every minute without adequate fluids could be causing irreparable harm to Kurt's organs.

The nurse felt that there were only a few minutes to contact the family before Kurt might die. She rushed down the hall to the nurse's station, pulled the chart for Kurt, and quickly dialed his son's phone number. Luckily the son answered and confirmed her advice to assist Kurt with intravenous infusion for hydration.

The nurse returned to the paramedics and was relieved to find Kurt still alive. She explained the family's request to assist Kurt, but the paramedics refused to act, saying that they wanted to speak with the son. The nurse insisted that they go ahead and give the intravenous until they could contact Kurt's son again. The young paramedic would not allow further medical measures until he spoke with the son himself.

It seemed like an eternity for the paramedic to walk down the hall, confirm the conversation with the son, and return to Kurt's bedside. The intravenous was finally started. The nurse knew that Kurt's heart could stop any minute, and she prayed that it was not too late. She also knew that the paramedics surely would not do CPR because the POLST form indicated "no CPR." If the heart stopped, there would not be sufficient time for conversations with family to start CPR.

Kurt made it to the hospital for a short stay and was transferred to a hospice to complete his end-of-life experience. The doctors believed that he would not recover from this illness and expected that he would die within a week. However, after several weeks, Kurt recovered his good health and returned to the assisted living community.

After his return, the nurse saw Kurt with his hat and coat, standing at the front door, and inquired where he was going. He said that he was going to walk down to the physician's office to change the directions on his POLST form. The nurse was glad that she was able to serve as a health-care advocate for Kurt, because her quick actions saved his life and enabled him to enjoy many more years in good health.

Lenny Had More Life to Live

Sometimes the assisted living nurse serves as the advocate for the resident and the family members who need help navigating through health-care decisions.

Lenny lived at the assisted living community for four years. He was in his eighties and had moderate dementia with Parkinson's disease. In his younger years, he had been an engineer and enjoyed sailing. He knew everything about boats. Although he had not been in a boat for many years, any mention of a boat would bring on a smile from ear to ear. He loved to tell stories about his many sailing adventures, including sailing around the world.

Lenny had a regular daily routine. He went for long walks with his walker, sat at the same seat each day at meals with friends that he enjoyed, and participated in group activities. One morning, Lenny walked to the dining room with his walker, sat in the same seat to socialize with his usual friends, and ordered the usual "special" for breakfast. After he finished his breakfast, he got up to walk, became faint, and fell against the wall and down to the floor. The nurses assessed Lenny and noted that he was still conscious, but his blood pressure was very low. He was sent to the hospital with paramedics for evaluation.

Later that day, the nurse received a surprising call from Lenny's son, Kip. Kip was very upset, stating that the doctor felt that Lenny's quality of life was not worth preserving because of dementia. The emergency room doctor had found an infection that had caused the blood pressure to drop but recommended that Lenny should not receive antibiotics to treat the infection.

The doctor recommended that Lenny be moved to a hospice and allowed to die with comfort medications, as indicated on his POLST form.

Kip and the nurse discussed his father's quality of life. Despite Lenny's slight confusion and the recommendations listed in his POLST form, both the nurse and Kip felt that Lenny was happy in his daily routine and should be given antibiotics and a chance to continue with his life. Kip asked the nurse to speak with the doctor to advocate on Lenny's behalf.

The doctor did not agree with the nurse's request because of his perception that was influenced by the POLST form. He did not understand how Lenny could have a good quality of life with Parkinson's disease and moderate dementia. The doctor stated that if Lenny truly understood his condition, he probably would want to die peacefully rather than be treated for the infection.

The nurse realized that the doctor was not familiar with caring for aging adults with dementia. Therefore, she served as the advocate and explained to this doctor that there still could be a wonderful quality of life with this condition and much life to enjoy. As a result, the doctor agreed to discharge Lenny with an inexpensive antibiotic that cured the infection and preserved his life. Lenny enjoyed his routine for many more years, and Kip thanked the nurse for being an advocate for both his dad and him.

Later, when Lenny's condition suddenly declined, the POLST form was honored. In this situation, Kip knew that the POLST form would serve as a proper directive for his father's wishes.

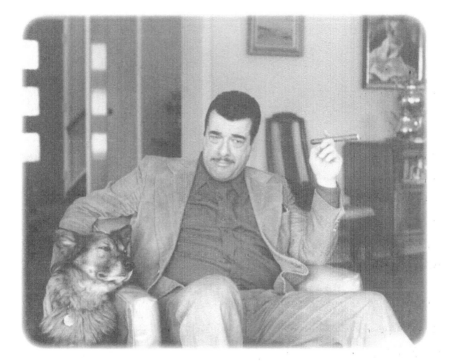

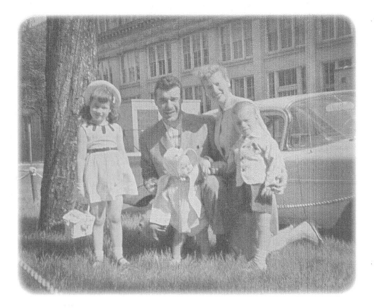

Chapter 9

Family Trials and Tribulations

M any of us have fond memories of our parents because we grew up with their loving care and guidance. Now it is our turn to care for Mom and Dad, with their declining health, because they are unable to lead independent lives. Although it may feel like an unwanted burden, many adult children are willing to accept this responsibility because they feel that they owe it to their parents or that it is their obligation.

Dealing with Guilt Feelings

In caring for their elderly parents, most people find themselves in uncharted territory and may feel hopeless. There may be frustration and guilt from feelings that they are not doing enough for Mom or Dad or they are not doing it correctly. Sometimes the guilt feelings arise in adult children who cannot care for their parents by themselves in their own homes. Such guilt feelings can cause adult children to blame staff members for not doing enough. These adult children can be overdemanding of staff as a reaction to their own inability to reconcile feelings of guilt.

"Mom and Dad once cared for me, so now it is my turn." It may seem that skills for raising children may be similar to those needed to take care of aging parents. However, these skills are not the same because the challenges are much different. Adult care is not the same as child care. Changing an adult diaper is far more unpleasant than changing the diaper for a toddler or infant. The elderly person is much bigger, and so is the mess. With adults who have Alzheimer's disease or other causes of dementia, the resistance to being changed from soiled clothes may be a great challenge, especially when there are associated feelings of humiliation. Mom was there for us as children, even when we threw tantrums. We seem to feel that it should be our obligation to change their diaper as easily as they changed ours, but this is not always the case.

A huge challenge in caring for the elderly may occur when it is time to bathe them. Many elderly people become very stiff and unable to climb into a tub or take a shower by themselves. Many elderly people have balance problems and require wall grips. It may be hard to give them a shower without finding yourself getting just as wet as them.

Another challenge in care of the elderly parent is realizing that Mom or Dad will forget things. They may require constant daily and hourly reminders or guidance. They may forget where they need to go next or where they put things, and they may even forget your identity. It could be an endless and exhausting cycle to get them through the day.

Surrendering the care of Mom or Dad to someone else can lead to feelings of inadequacy, ineptness, or guilt. Many times, these adult children develop endless and unrealistic expectations to replace the guilt they feel. They are emotionally unable to appreciate the care that is provided to their parents by someone else. They believe there is always more that the staff can do for their parents, and it should be more than what they can do themselves.

Adult children often have unrealistic expectations like having the care staff fix Mom's hair or makeup exactly how she used to do it herself. If it is not done correctly, they may blame themselves because of their perceived failure to find the proper care. They may blame themselves if Mom does not appear the same as they remember when she lived at home.

It is unpleasant to be overwhelmed with these guilt feelings. Many times, Mom or Dad may be unaware of the sacrifices their children are making for them. If they were aware of the reality of how their family members were caring for and coordinating their needs, they would believe they raised them properly and would be proud.

Adrianna's Fight for Perfection

Adrianna was an only child who struggled with the guilt feelings of being unable to care for her mother, Hilda, in her home. Adrianna was married and had two teenage children. Her husband, John, traveled a lot for business, and Adrianna enjoyed traveling with him.

Hilda was very demanding and insisted on perfection. Adrianna kept the home in very good order, but she struggled with feelings that her efforts could never live up to her mother's expectations. Adrianna always had perfectly fixed hair, was immaculately dressed in the latest fashions, and kept a spotless house in perfect order. She devoted her life to keeping every aspect of her family life in perfect control.

Adrianna did not attempt to care for Hilda at her own home because of her travel schedule and her fear of a negative effect on her marriage and children. After she placed Hilda in the assisted living community, Adrianna felt tremendous relief that her mother was being cared for, but she also felt tremendous guilt that she was unable to accommodate Hilda in her own home.

Adrianna came to eat lunch with her mother every day, and she had endless requests that stemmed from her guilt feelings about not taking care of her mother herself. Adrianna complained that Hilda's makeup was not applied exactly as in her portrait, the earrings were not the correct match for her outfit, or her watch was not set to the correct minute. Many tiny and endless demands would be listed after each visit.

Adrianna took her mother away for a long weekend to a family wedding and provided all aspects of her mother's care. On her return from the weekend, Adrianna was a changed person. Adrianna took staff aside and thanked them for aspects of care that she was unable to accomplish on the weekend outing.

During her visits with Hilda, Adrianna began to overlook issues of imperfection and realized that her mother was cared for in the best way possible. Although Adrianna continued to have guilt feelings, she became more accepting of the assisted living situation and realized that it was as perfect as it could be for her.

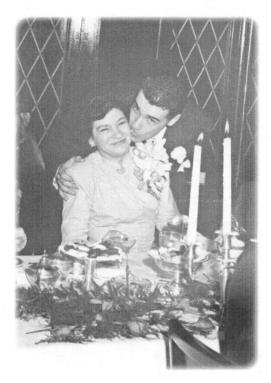

No Limit to a Son's Love

Tom's guilt feelings came from his inability to cure all his mother's ailments—an unrealistic goal. Tom loved his mother, Edith, very much. He placed her in the assisted living community where she would be in a higher care setting, with more staff and professional nurse supervision.

Edith had respiratory issues and required oxygen, and she needed assistance with dressing. However, she had no memory loss or decline. Although Edith was happy with every aspect of service and care in the assisted living setting, Tom was never satisfied because he saw his mother's health continue to decline. Tom complained regardless of how much care was given to Edith, whether the care was necessary or simply from kindness.

Tom visited during dinners, and he usually ordered several courses of menu items for his mother because he was displeased with what she was being served. He remembered food preferences from Edith's past and insisted that she try them all. Edith did not have the same appetite as in the past, and food tasted less appealing to her because of her illness. She was content with what was served and said nothing about Tom's excessive ordering because she knew that he meant well.

When Tom was at home, he used to call the assisted living front desk, frantic that his mother needed help. He would say that he had just spoken with her on the telephone, and she was short of breath. Staff members would drop everything and run up to Edith's apartment, only to find her resting without any shortness of breath or need of assistance. Edith would question why we were coming in to check on her. Tom's dissatisfaction and complaints were endless, even though her care was complete. However, her health continued to deteriorate.

The doctors were unable to cure Edith's chronic condition, and eventually she was placed on hospice services. Tom's demands on staff members continued to grow as Edith's health situation declined. Staff members realized that they were frequently caring more for Tom's guilt than Edith's health-care needs. This unfortunate situation stemmed from his guilt feelings that could not be resolved or minimized.

Tom came to terms with his guilt feelings when he had open conversations with staff members that allowed him to share his feelings of helplessness. After Edith passed away, Tom felt relief, and he accepted her declining health and death. He understood that there was nothing more he could do, and he had to let go of the situation.

Feelings of Love and Hate

It is healthy and normal for grown children to have strong emotions about the declining health of elderly parents. There are intense, deep-seated feelings within adult children because of the genetic relationship and codependent nurturing roles with their parents. People who seem well adjusted and functional in their daily lives can "fall to pieces" when they express feelings about their parents. Many people have their own intense feelings about a dominant father or mother who has an overbearing personality.

We may have disappointments about why Mom or Dad could not do certain things differently or behave better, but we may realize that perhaps they did the best they could. Many people struggle and seek to make sense of a relationship with a parent that was not ideal.

The best way to approach these intense feelings is to acknowledge that the conflicts exist and learn what they represent. Do you feel love, hate, or resentment? Some people choose to resolve this with or without therapists who might help sort through these emotions. Accept the fact that it is normal to have strong feelings, such as deep-seated hatred.

Many people feel that they may be criticized when they reveal that they have intense feelings, such as hatred or anger because of unresolved parental situations from the past. Despite judgment or criticism from others, it is best to acknowledge and accept our own feelings and move forward. With complete acceptance of feelings, it becomes possible to break the chain of unwanted child-rearing behaviors that can be passed to future generations.

It can take tremendous inner strength to accept feelings that originate from childhood relationships with Mom or Dad. These feelings and situations may have developed over a long time, and it may require time to get beyond them. Many adult children are not confronted with the reality of their deep-seated feelings for Mom and Dad until they must care from them. Adult children may not be prepared emotionally to address this complex situation of unresolved feelings.

Mom and Dad, in their present state of memory loss, cannot validate the feelings of their adult children because they may not remember past experiences. Dad may not remember his breakfast or the identity of the adult child, and the adult child frequently must deal with these memories alone. Dad with dementia lives in the present moment, and whatever happened in the past must be reconciled alone, without Dad's help.

As a nurse and caregiver, I always emphasize to adult children that I may care for your dad, but I cannot rectify issues between a parent and adult child. These issues must be addressed independent of the alternative care situation outside the home, and they include three components:

1. Past memories of the parent
2. The present relationship with the parent
3. The turmoil that the adult children carry within themselves

Adult children must put aside unresolved feelings when Dad has dementia and focus on his safety and health care. Dad is in a vulnerable position of need, and the adult child must focus on the daily coordination of care. The reality is that the world of dementia makes no sense, and this is not the same person you knew as a child and most of your adult years.

Skeletons in the Closet

It is important to connect with your parents to discuss unresolved feelings. When the opportunity arises, capture the moment because the opportunity may never return. A moment of clarity may occur at the beginning of Dad's memory loss, and this may be the last chance for a coherent conversation. In this last sliver of time in your relationship, you have a chance to allow them to tell "their story." This may clarify aspects of the past and present and improve understanding between your parents and you.

Questions that many ask in these last-chance situations are:

» What was your childhood like?

» What did you really do in the war?

» How did you feel about me being born and about raising me?

All these questions are the beginning of very meaningful conversations that you will carry with you, long after Dad has passed on. You might want to explore how Mom and Dad feel by asking other "coming to terms" or "icebreaker" questions, such as:

» Are the "golden years" what you thought they would be?

» How do you feel about death?

» What happens to people when they die?

It can be great when Dad takes on his part of reconciling past occurrences, to understand and clarify situations, or just listen. However, most often he will not respond as you wish he would, and you must settle for your positive efforts of trying to make the connection. The meaning you gather in last conversations can be a gift. Sometimes it is comforting to clarify how you feel and tell Dad your thoughts.

A Voice Finally Heard

Clare was persistent in her efforts to have her father open up so she could understand situations in her life with him. Clare had a very rocky relationship with her dad. He had been in and out of the hospital frequently, each time miraculously defying death. Clare had attempted conversations with him many times, but he did not relate or converse about anything meaningful.

Clare felt a huge amount of hate, love, and confusion toward her dad. One day, she was so overwhelmed with the unresolved past that she drove the hour and a half to her dad and sat with him until all was said. While he lay in the hospital, she sat at his bedside and shared her frustration about his not opening up to her. She spilled her feelings about the times he hurt her, deserted her, and was never there when she needed him. Tears streamed down her face as she poured out a lifetime of memories of anger and frustration.

In the end, she looked up at her dad, who was staring at her with an attentive stone face. He leaned over, hugged her, and said, "I'm sorry." For the first time in Clare's life, he acknowledged his faults. He died months later, but Clare was satisfied that she had a chance to connect with him in a meaningful way. This experience of sharing her feelings with him helped her start to put the past behind her and move on.

Not Able to Forgive

Drake was a resident at the assisted living community. He was a hardworking doctor before his retirement. He was home very little because of his long workday, but he supported his wife and three children financially. He had a history of drinking alcohol; although he was never diagnosed as an alcoholic, his drinking caused occasional emotional outbursts with family members.

One day, he was the driver of a vehicle and was involved in a fatal accident that caused the death of one of his children. The details of the accident were unclear, but it was never established that he was under the influence of alcohol. Drake could never forgive himself. When he moved to the assisted living community, his family ignored him. They paid for his assisted living care but never called or visited. Nurses from the assisted living community called Drake's family with updates, but family members were not interested in him under any circumstance. His family members were still angry with him, blaming him for the death of his child in the car accident years ago. The family members refused to forgive, and they did not return calls from staff members. Eventually, Drake died alone, without any family present.

If the family members can ever reconcile their feelings and come to terms with the fatal car crash, it will be too late to say good-bye to Drake.

The Jilted Sibling

Each adult child views her childhood experience as unique and different from that of her siblings, even in the same household. Sometimes these perceptions create feelings that "Mom always loved the other sibling more," "she never did anything for me," or "I had it the hardest." However, in caring for elderly parents, families fare better when they move past these squabbles and come together.

Rachel, in her eighties, had two daughters who continued their childhood behaviors of competing for Mom's attention, despite their adult years. When Rachel was in the assisted living community under their shared responsibility, the sisters became very competitive with each other about who could give the most attention to their mother and who could be more responsible in directing Mom's care with the staff. One sister directed staff members with one approach to incontinent care for Rachel, and then the other sister redirected the care differently. This jealous situation, with each daughter vying for attention by controlling aspects of Rachel's care, continued until Rachel showed favor to one or wanted attention from the other. When Rachel showed attention to one daughter, the other daughter felt left out and abandoned.

The two sisters planned their visits when the other sibling was not there, to avoid direct conflict and to get Mom's full attention and approval. Holiday family events were challenging to coordinate because each daughter wanted her own time with Mom. When a photographer came for family portraits, Rachel had two portraits taken, one with each daughter separate from the other, because the daughters refused to have one sitting with all the family together.

Rachel was aware of her children's conflict with each other and their separation. After years of unsuccessful efforts, she gave up trying to bring her children together. Finally, after Rachel developed kidney failure and was close to death, she was able to push her daughters to call a truce.

The assisted living community and other alternative care environments will not help families resolve their deep-seated past issues and behaviors. It is up to the adult children themselves to resolve their issues and move past these feelings and behavior patterns carried over from childhood.

It is difficult for some adult children to put the past to rest and realize that there are current and more important issues with Mom or Dad now in dependent care.

The Odd Family Member

Many families have a member who is different from the others and does not fit in. This can cause challenges in situations when the family must pull together. When family members disagree about care, health-care providers must follow directives given by the person who has power of attorney.

In extreme cases, the majority of family members may disregard the odd one and treat that person as an outcast. For the staff in any alternative care setting, the family member with the power of attorney is the decision maker, even if this person is the odd family member. Assisted living staff members use the term "odd family member syndrome" when there are disagreements and turmoil between family members during the decision-making process.

The odd family member may not appear for many years. This happened with Willy, a resident for five years in the assisted living community. His son, Don, who was a loving son and reasonable person, held the power of attorney for his father. Don occasionally visited his father and told us about five other siblings. When

Willy's health was fading, the siblings seemed to be in agreement. However, Lana from California appeared. She was the "odd family member," and she gave different instructions, causing upset, added confusion, and delayed decision making. When the other siblings learned that Lana had called, it was as if an emotional explosion had occurred within the family, signaling to the staff that the odd family member had surfaced.

When this happens, family members address the situation best when they:

>   confront or approach the odd family member directly to avoid delays in treating Mom or Dad;

>   do not avoid the person, because that may aggravate behavioral issues;

>   advise the staff members not to get mixed messages from the odd family member, so proper decisions are made when there are disagreements;

>   do not allow her to go directly to health-care providers because this may cause confusion among physicians, health-care providers, and staff members providing care.

Another challenging family situation arises when one family member is seeking financial gain or assistance. This family member may visit to have the parent in the assisted living community take him to lunch or give him money. The "odd family member" may drain Mom or Dad financially as expenses accumulate and seem endless.

The odd family member may have financial power of attorney, either alone or jointly with another sibling. This family outcast may acquire a lavish lifestyle while the parent under care is quickly running low on funds. Parents designate who will be in charge of their financial and health-care affairs, and this may occur long before problems develop in relationships within the family. The odd family member, spending all of Mom or Dad's money, may quickly create an adverse situation within the family, resulting in legal battles that add to the stressful financial situation.

A Sibling's Battle

Kate and Don had joint power of attorney for their mother's affairs. Kate had her mom in our assisted living community for several years. Kate lived close by and handled most financial and health matters. Kate called to tell us when her brother, Don, would be visiting because she did not want him to be alone with his mother. Don used to write out checks for his mother to sign, payable to himself, or have the mother go to lunch or shop with him and have her pay.

Don was financially stressed and careless with his mother's money. Although Kate's attempt to control her brother's spending was stressful, her openness with the assisted living personnel helped minimize his behavior. By communicating with the staff, Kate limited her brother's behavior without a legal battle.

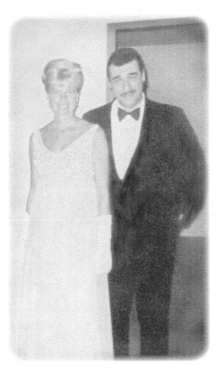

The Dementia Divorce

Many elderly people remain in long-term marriages but realize that these relationships did not provide long-term "marital bliss." As they reflect on their marriage of fifty or sixty years, they may recall long periods when love was missing, and they may have difficulty remembering the happy moments that interspersed times of turmoil.

Long-term marriages evolve with time. Parents with children may grow apart and decide to separate or divorce. Although some people grow closer after the kids have left the nest, the children may be the primary thread that holds the marriage together. Marriages can readjust in different ways after the children leave home. Some couples reconnect to find the love and partnership that they once had before the children arrived.

With other couples, the marriage may evolve to a congenial

partnership in which the partners age together and support each other in a manner similar to roommates. These spouses may argue and irritate each other when they cross boundaries, but they stay together because they prefer this more than the inconveniences of separation. They co-exist as "marriage roommates," helping each other and doing no more or less than what is necessary to maintain the relationship. They create a balance of "give and take" that works for them, enjoying the joint family connections with their children, grandchildren, and family events.

This partnership marriage can continue for many years until a change in circumstance occurs and disrupts the balanced responsibilities to each other. This change may occur when one partner's health declines and he needs more help from the other partner. One elderly parent elevates his level of responsibility and becomes the caretaker of the other. The balance in the relationship is shifted, and the added responsibility may be unwanted by the partner who becomes the caretaker. This burden of one partner taking care of the other may be stressful to the relationship, prompting the caretaker to seek help from an alternative care setting, such as an assisted living community.

The caretaker spouse may remain at home after placing the declining spouse into the care setting. I refer to this physical separation in long-term marriages as the "dementia divorce." It is the physical separation of two elderly married people, with no legal divorce on paper, that occurs because of their personal circumstances. This may occur with other diseases, but dementia is the most common reason for this type of health-related physical separation of married people.

There may be some very special and long-term marriages that continue because of deep-seated love and respect for each other. These fairy-tale marriages are rare, but they do exist, with intense love that persists after many years. These "still in love" long-term marriages are not immune to the dementia divorce.

Even in these very connected marriages of love, many spouses who provide care become exhausted. When the demands for care are beyond what they can personally provide, they must place their partner in an alternative care environment.

The dementia divorce also occurs when the stress of being the caretaker is so great that it causes a decline of the caretaker's health. It is in the best interest of the caretakers to preserve their health and have the spouse in need of care move to an alternative environment. The committed caretaker may resist saving themselves because they are committed to the marriage vows that had not addressed the extreme duress of taking care of their declining spouse.

The caretaker spouse willingly and lovingly assumes the care of the spouse and accepts the daily sacrifices and limitations in their own lives to provide needed care to their spouse. However, the caretakers often:

» don't eat properly,

» endure sleepless nights,

» become physically and emotionally drained from taking care of their spouse,

» find the experience detrimental to their own health and well-being.

When the caretaker has a health crisis, the family is forced to intervene and come to the rescue. If the caretaker is not protected from the responsibility of providing care beyond his abilities, he may end up in the hospital with stress-related health issues. Frequently, even after sixty years of marriage, the caretaker may be relieved that he no longer has this burden of care. The exhausted spouse is grateful that somebody else initiated the separation of care that they felt was taboo.

Adult children may be surprised that the caretaker parent will remove herself from contact so quickly. The adult children may remember challenging times between their married parents, but they had not experienced them in a physical separation. This physical separation of the parents places additional responsibility on the adult children to help with the parent who needs care.

Resentment Builds

Some elderly people resent spending their "golden years" in retirement with the new responsibility of caring for their spouse. They experience anger and frustration, and they blame the declining spouse for the situation. When a caretaker spouse harbors such negative feelings, it is difficult for him or her to step into a caregiver role with compassion.

The caregiver may reflect on the past, when the spouse was unfaithful or was emotionally or physically abusive. The caregiver may still harbor bad feelings, which add to the anger and resentment of having to provide care. When past emotional issues surface, it may be difficult for the healthier spouse to assume the obligation and sacrifice of providing the care. The care provided is more abusive than loving.

When the adult children observe that Mom and Dad are in a dysfunctional relationship, with one spouse being neglectful in caring for the other, the children must take charge. They may initiate the "dementia divorce" separation by placing one parent in an alternative care environment and keeping the other parent at home, away from care responsibilities.

Despite close involvement and concern, the adult children may be unable to provide the support required to avoid their parents having a "dementia divorce." Previously, the children were the key focus for Mom and Dad; however, they currently live very separate lives and may have limited time and resources to provide care. Furthermore, Mom and Dad may be concerned about their grown children's life situations and may not want to burden their children by asking for help. The parents may pretend that everything is fine to avoid troubling the children. As a result, adult children may be unaware of the care requirements for Mom or Dad until the situation has deteriorated and has become too difficult to correct at home.

Long-Term Marriages

The situations that cause dementia divorce may be especially prevalent with the generation of people currently in their seventies or older. The long-term marriages of fifty to sixty years that characterize that generation may create coexisting situations that lead to the dementia divorce. Many people of that generation believe that a marriage should not be broken under any circumstance. They were told to stay married despite abuse, financial crisis, problems with children, or illness. They viewed these situations as included in their vows that stated, "Until death do us part." Therefore, the only way to separate physically may occur when health needs decline and one spouse must be moved to a care community. This separation is both physical and emotional, and there may be no potential to reconstruct the marriage that Mom and Dad had in the past.

Peg's Last Straw

Rick was married to Peg, and they had four grown children. Rick was a demanding father and husband and had a successful career as an engineer. When Rick's family and wife, Peg, brought him to our assisted living community, we admitted him directly from the hospital. He was in very poor condition, confused, and weak. He had bruises and open wounds from repeated falls.

Rick had lived at home with Peg for sixty-five years. It was not a loving relationship; it was a marriage of obligation. Now Rick needed care, and Peg could not give more of herself. Peg had much resentment toward Rick from their long-term strained relationship, and she could not do anything more than the bare minimum. Rick's decline resulted from Peg's inability to care for him. The family was unaware of how poorly Rick had been eating or how many times he had fallen. Eventually, Rick ate something that made him so confused that he fell and sustained an injury that led to hospitalization.

This fall was the crisis that led Rick's children to intervene and separate Rick and Peg. After Rick moved to the assisted living community, Peg pulled herself away in a "dementia divorce," neither visiting nor calling. The busy children made few visits, except for one daughter, Trish. Although Trish had not been involved previously, she became the only family member who took responsibility for assisting with the partnership in care.

Protecting Emma

The dementia divorce may be initiated by the adult children to protect one of the parents from potential harm. For Vince and Emma, who had been married for sixty years, the three grown children intervened to protect Emma.

Vince had a successful career in commercial development and a previous military career. He had an abrasive personality his entire life, including a militant approach to raising the children. As Vince aged with progressing dementia, his abrasive personality became increasingly more visible, and he was unable to contain his rage. Vince directed most of his rage toward Emma because she was the closest person to him, but she could not tolerate the emotional outbursts. Emma attempted to counter the verbal outbursts by arguing back or leaving the house.

The emotional outbursts became worse and progressed to physical rage. Vince threw items and occasionally grabbed and physically threatened Emma. Although Vince loved Emma and had no intention of hurting her, he could not control himself because of the dementia; he had lost the emotional tools that enabled him to remain calm.

One evening, the three adult children were called to the home because Vince was uncontrollable. He was violent and had hurt Emma. He had grabbed her and pushed her to the ground. The children initiated a dementia divorce to protect Emma. Vince was taken to an adult-care setting and put on medication to assist him with his emotions. With medication treatment, he was able to contain his outbursts, but Emma did not want him to return home.

Vince could not remember the events of the argument because of his dementia. He felt that it was a small argument that should have been forgiven the next day. He felt rejected by Emma and became very depressed. He was put on antidepressant drugs to assist with the depression, but each day he waited at the door, hoping his wife would forgive him and bring him home. Emma neither visited nor called because she feared that Vince would harm her.

Vince remained at the assisted living community and died. At the funeral service, the family spoke of Vince without mentioning his decline with dementia. They remarked that he was a giving husband and father. Emma spoke of her husband, Vince, in a loving and caring way. For this family, there was no lack of love, and there was no dysfunctional relationship. The dementia divorce was established for Emma's safety because of Vince's decline with Alzheimer's disease.

Susan's New Love

The fairy-tale loving relationship is not immune to the dementia divorce. Susan and Robert were married sixty-six years, and they had grown children. Susan was quickly declining with dementia, and Robert had been caring for her for more than a year. He realized that Susan's care was progressing beyond his capability.

Robert moved himself and his declining wife into a one-bedroom apartment in our assisted living community. He continued to care for her with our help until it became too much for him, even in that setting. Eventually, Susan was moved to the higher memory care area, and Robert stayed in the minimal assistance area of the community to be near her. Every day, he visited and helped care for her.

Eventually, Susan did not recognize Robert as her husband. She paired up with another man in the dementia unit, holding his hand and sitting with him when she could. Robert continued to come as frequently as possible to assist with her care, even though Susan frequently was with another man.

Susan's dementia led to an emotional separation and dementia divorce because she did not recognize Robert as her husband. To her, he became just another person providing care to her. Robert may have been hurt by Susan's connection with another man, but he never voiced any emotional pain. He continued to care for Susan and love her as he vowed to do in their marriage. Susan died with Robert sitting by her side until her last breath.

CHAPTER 10

The Assisted Living Community— Help beyond Home

Alternative care for people with dementia may include group homes, nursing homes, in-home options, and assisted living communities. An assisted living community or other senior care residence should provide Dad with adequate care in a safe, monitored environment. It can be difficult to find the right place for Dad because there are many options. The adult children want him to have excellent care in a place where he will enjoy living. Dad usually does not remember the turmoil that led to the decision to place him in a long-term environment away from home. Dad does not understand the stress and worry that he has caused his spouse and family because of his memory loss or increased health-care needs.

Dad believes and expects that his spouse or family will be with him or visit soon. The telephone may become Dad's lifeline to his missing family. He may use the telephone repeatedly each day, attempting to connect with them. The time of day is meaningless to him. He may call his family at all hours of the day and night. The calls may be excessive and exhausting for family members who have guilt feelings that they are not caring for Dad at home.

Assisted living staff may recommend that families have caller identification and voicemail, and the family may screen Dad's frequent calls to minimize disruption. Dad with dementia is waiting to go home to be with his spouse, and he does not understand the reason for the change. Regardless of what he is told, he is lost because his short-term memory is gone. The long-term memories of living at home and his daily routines that include his family members still prevail in his mind.

The caregivers in the assisted living community repeatedly redirect Dad from the front door and telephone. This may continue for many weeks until Dad eventually adapts to his new environment without his family. Dad is confused and believes that the past is still the present. He may insist on going to work, paying bills, or participating in other daily routines from his past.

In the early stages of dementia, Dad may respond to redirection with sadness and frustration because he may realize that he is forgetting. As the dementia progresses, he will not understand the extent of his memory loss and may become frustrated and angry.

Entering the World of Dementia

It may be difficult for the caregivers and family of a person with dementia to address undesirable behaviors when he or she moves into an assisted living community. A useful method includes trying to understand how he or she views the world. If Dad believes that he is living his life of forty to fifty years earlier, we might go back to that time to understand his behavior. Rationality does not work for patients with dementia because they are not capable of understanding reality. It would be analogous to communicating with a toddler and trying to explain a complicated concept that is beyond his comprehension. The adult must be managed differently than a young child, because the adult is aware of his adult age and believes that he has more wisdom. If the distorted view of reality is ignored and not managed properly, the emotions and undesirable behaviors can escalate and get out of control.

Unwanted behavior can be avoided by using creativity. One assisted living resident had undesirable emotional outbursts about his missing wife, until I placed a "Welcome" sign on his door that included his wife's name. He did not believe that his wife had passed away, and he did not remember attending her funeral the previous summer. By seeing both his and her names on the "Welcome" sign, he felt comfortable and had no more undesirable outbursts.

Another resident insisted on going home, but the home no longer existed. I repeatedly went through the motions of calling a limousine service for his transport "home," and he always changed his mind about leaving when he was told about the high cost of the limousine service.

With another resident who wanted to leave, I "waited for the bus" with him until he gave up because the bus never arrived. There was no actual bus stop where we waited.

In another case, the resident wanted to call his family, but the family members had requested that they not be called. Therefore, I went through the motions of making repeated calls, using phone numbers that I knew would be busy or have no answer. The appearance of making an effort to satisfy his request was reassuring for him, even though we had no success reaching a family member. He simply wanted to know that someone was listening to him and following his orders.

Within one month or less, Dad usually adapts to his new environment. He may become familiar with the new routine in the assisted living setting. With time, he usually will acclimate to the new environment and other people. Residents in the assisted living community get to know each other, develop relationships, and become supportive of each other. The staff members and other residents eventually replace their family and friends, who are no longer present. A community develops between residents as they become familiar with one another. They can identify changes in the behavior of other residents, even if they themselves have memory impairment or dementia. With the help of other residents, the unfamiliar environment becomes friendlier and feels more like home.

Collette's Connection

Collette had moderate dementia, and she was always waiting for her parents to come for her. She had lived in the assisted living community for more than two years, but she had forgotten that this was her home. She became acquainted with Kurt, a fellow assisted living resident. Kurt was more alert than Collette, but he talked with her frequently because he enjoyed her company.

Kurt developed a serious infection and was hospitalized. When he returned to the assisted living community, he was much more confused than before. He did not remember what he had to do or where to go. He did not know his location, the reason he was at the community, or his family's location.

Despite her own state of dementia, Collette noticed that Kurt had declined and that he needed help and comfort. She could not remember his name, but she knew that they had routinely interacted. Collette called to Kurt across the lobby. Kurt strolled over to her, confused, and he asked her if she knew the whereabouts of his family. He was happy that she took an interest in him, hoping she knew more about his situation.

Collette instructed him to sit down next to her, and he did exactly as she said. She looked at him caringly, and she told him not to worry and that she would watch over him. She then reached over and held his hand, and they sat in silence together. Despite her own situation, Collette was able to recognize when someone else was in need. She was willing to help Kurt, and at that moment, she was like family to him.

The Business of Assisted Living

The assisted living industry is growing rapidly and may continue to expand because of the aging baby boomer population. Assisted living communities vary widely in level of service, each attempting to address the care of the elderly in different stages of decline. Some communities simply provide an independent setting with minimal assistance, meals, and basic "checking in" for Mom. Other communities are equipped to focus on high-level, hands-on assistance in all aspects of care, including meals and snacks.

The simpler assisted living communities include basic units, called apartments, a common dining area, and additional areas for residents to sit and relax or socialize. The more lavish assisted living communities can be mistaken for five-star hotels and may include several restaurants or eating areas, theaters, hair salons, and ballrooms for parties and other events. Most communities are paid privately and very costly, but the right place that follows through on promises will be worth every cent paid.

The Care Placement Decision: Whom Can We Trust?

When the time comes to search for care options for Mom, it may be difficult to know where to start and whom to trust. The decision about Mom's care community includes these considerations:

» Does this care community meet Mom's current and long-term physical needs?

» Is the place a good match for Mom's emotional needs? Does it feel like home? Will it be comfortable for her?

» Will this care situation effectively address Mom's safety concerns?

» Does Mom's financial portfolio support this option?

The most reliable people to find the best care option for Mom are the people who know her, care about her, and love her. These individuals will most likely put their hearts and souls into researching the many care options for the elderly and find the best place for her. These trusted individuals may be family members, friends, or legal guardians, assigned by a court of law, who have an obligation to do their best. Mom may have previously and legally assigned the role of decision maker for her care situation to a health-care power of attorney. The authority of the health-care power of attorney usually is limited to health-care issues, and this individual must work in partnership with the legally assigned financial power of attorney to find the best place for Mom.

Ella's Bargain

Ella was an elderly lady who was experiencing memory decline. In her early stages of forgetfulness, she was aware of the memory loss and realized that she needed a plan for the future. Her husband had died several years earlier, and she had nobody to care for her: no siblings, no friends, and no relatives.

Ella knew a young couple, neighbors who were interested in her property. Therefore, she made a contract deal with these neighbors. The neighbors agreed to coordinate Ella's care in an alternative care environment until her death, and then they would inherit her land. The young couple gladly accepted the responsibility of care for Ella because of the benefit of receiving her land that they desired, but they did not have any love or compassion for Ella. Ella chose the assisted living community where I worked, but as her condition worsened, she could not recognize others and was unaware of daily happenings.

The neighbors had been appointed by Ella as having power of attorney, and they assumed the direction of Ella's care, based on the signed contract with Ella. However, Ella's neighbors were not interested in her well-being, and they had signed the contract to help with her care only to receive her land. They did not return telephone calls and did not help with hospital or doctor visits. They became a hindrance to Ella's care, rather than a benefit, because they refused to allow her to go to the hospital, did not agree to anything that would improve her health, and did not pay the bills. Eventually, Ella had to move to a nursing home where there were more resources available, such as social workers and legal contacts, to address this unusual circumstance.

Unfortunately, when Ella made this care arrangement with her neighbors several years earlier, she did not understand the importance of love and true compassion in the responsibility of her care. Ella had made a wrong assumption, believing incorrectly that a financial gain for her neighbors would inspire them to behave as caring and compassionate individuals and provide responsible guidance in her care.

The Care Staff Becomes Family

A family that is concerned about Mom will seek an assisted living community where Mom will receive excellent care. The family usually wants care equivalent in quality to their own care, had that been possible. In the assisted living community, we attempt to create an environment of care that a family can trust.

The loving and caring environment in an assisted living community is created by a collective effort of a team of special individuals. These special care staff members must have giving qualities that enable them to succeed with loving care. The caring staff member sets a great example and inspires the entire care staff team to do the same. The care team works together to collectively address Mom's needs more effectively than a single individual. The team addresses the issue of Mom asking the same question every five minutes, or her needing physically demanding help that would be too difficult for a single staff member. The staff team may consider alternating the individual staff member who will best address each task at any time.

In any alternative care environment, such as the assisted living community, there are many different levels of responsibility in the care of the elderly. The administrator or nurse will guide the entire team taking care of Mom or Dad. The team may need coaching and support to provide the highest level of care daily. It may require time to understand the resident's health-care issues. The team requires proper guidance to improve efficiency and support for each other in caring for the elderly.

When searching for an alternative living community for Mom or Dad, it is helpful to ask care staff members how long they have been employed at the care community. Long-term employees typically have more experience and are more attuned to elderly needs.

Beyond Bricks and Mortar

Families must evaluate the caring environment beyond the aesthetics of the beautiful building. The alternative care environment can appear beautiful to the observer, but the truly important challenge is to create a loving and caring home for Mom or Dad. Successful alternative care communities hire excellent staff that can connect with the other care members in positive ways.

To provide the best care, the community administrator must recognize the limitations and assets of the care staff. The administrator must place the staff members in situations that require their innate strengths and personal passions. The most difficult and important challenge for the administrator is to assign the best person to the most appropriate team and set of tasks. The administrator must identify and recruit the correct individuals who can excel and provide quality care. There may be successes and failures in hiring staff members, and some individuals may cause disappointment. The ultimate goal in hiring care staff is to find workers who provide compassion, love, and a caring environment for Mom or Dad.

Having the Right Stuff

How can adult children identify the best individuals for the care team—people who are capable of instituting proper and best practices? Who has the right stuff to be a care provider?

When evaluating an alternative care community for Mom or Dad, the first step is to meet the administrator or owner of the community. It is important to find the right people to create the foundation for care-based service, and this starts at the top. The tone and standards for the community are set by the leader, who is the administrator of the assisted living community or owner of the adult family or group home. The adult children may evaluate the leader's experience and knowledge about health-care and administrative issues. Any deficiencies in this area may be a "red flag" about possible limitations in experience or knowledge in the entire team.

The person in charge usually has the most knowledge of all staff members. Therefore, administrators usually do not hire anybody with more experience or credentials than themselves. Furthermore, potential staff members typically search for work under a boss who has higher qualifications or more experience than themselves. It could be frustrating for an employee to work under a boss who has less experience than the employee.

Qualities of a Qualified Administrator

A qualified administrator in charge of an assisted living community will pass down his or her knowledge and experience to the staff members and direct the success of the community. It is surprising that many people commit money and a beloved family member to an assisted living community without meeting the top administrator. This meeting is an important part of evaluating the overall community and will provide clues to determine whether or not the community is a proper fit for Mom or Dad.

There are several key qualities that families should evaluate when meeting the administrator or owner of a care community.

1. **Professionalism.** Professional appearance, good communication skills, and respect for others are qualities that carry over to the care provided and the community operation.

2. **Appropriate experience.** Does the administrator have a college degree or any quality care experience that is relevant to the care of Mom or Dad? Some individuals are very basically trained and open a care community without a much needed foundation of knowledge. Some care communities may hire newly graduated registered nurses (RNs) who have no experience in elderly care, primarily to claim that they employ a nurse. Some states have administrator certifications, but other states may allow administrators to come from business backgrounds, without any health-care experience. However, an alternative care community is a specialized health-care operation.

3. **Sense of purpose.** Select a manager who works in assisted living with a sense of purpose, to create a positive environment and provide excellent care. A manager who is solely concerned about financial profits, and who is not committed to the mission to provide elderly care, will set a poor example to the rest of the staff. Administrators who work in the assisted living business primarily to earn profits typically are task-oriented and impersonal; in their communities, the personal care is not done with any passion, the residents are unhappy with their care, and the staff members are frustrated. Poor leadership may be reflected in a high frequency of staff members calling in sick and a high staff turnover rate.

4. **Community or team culture.** The care team in an assisted living community develops a team culture specific to that community. New managers and staff who join an experienced team should know if they will be a good fit.

The staff members connect to form their own standards of care that provide a unique work environment. Tension and conflict may occur when a team member is not connected with the others on the team, making it difficult to complete the work. This may cause frustration because of a lack of team effort and satisfactory accomplishments in the job. The lack of a supportive community culture causes poor performance and higher staff turnover.

Hiring the Right Staff in Alternative Care Communities

Families frequently ask why there is so much staff turnover in the care environment. Hiring the right person in care-related jobs for the elderly population is a huge challenge for any administrator. It is difficult to find suitable staff members to care for people in declining health with memory loss. These jobs frequently pay below-average wages, and this limits the applicant pool.

The staff member must have passion for giving to others without expecting gratitude or monetary reward. During interviews, I tell potential employees that they will be working very hard. The rewards they receive will not be earned from their hourly wage, but from their personal accomplishments in caring for others.

An administrator may perform many interviews and check multiple references and personality profiles, but less than 50 percent of applicants will pass the screening requirements. At times, hiring the right person may seem to be a gamble, even if the person has a good résumé, telephone interview, references, and personal interview. The staff member may have a short period of employment because of limited skills.

Elderly care requires a complex mix of qualities to be successful, and these may be difficult to judge adequately during the interview. The most important qualities include sincerity, compassion, caring, and patience. The most successful candidates are those who work from their hearts. These special people are primarily motivated by a passion to give and help others, not by financial reward. It is difficult to describe these qualities adequately within the job description, and it frequently requires good luck to find the suitable employee.

Ken, a twenty-five-year-old marketing director, had the responsibility of hiring the concierges in the assisted living community. He hired only young, inexperienced staff who did not complete their tasks at work. Eventually, Ken was replaced by Daisy, who was more professional. After several months, it was evident that the employees hired by Daisy were of much higher quality. They were hard workers who could perform the tasks in their job position, and they respected Daisy as an example of high job performance.

Candidates from other industries occasionally apply for positions in an elderly care setting. Many want a change and look forward to the opportunity to help others. These individuals sometimes have made good incomes in their past professions, and they desire to enter a more meaningful career path and contribute personally to others. These people are typically great employees because they are not in the caring profession for the "almighty dollar." These employees who change careers must learn the workings of health care, but their success comes from compassion, a sense of purpose, and a desire to contribute to others.

As the administrator, most caregivers I have hired are culturally diverse, from many different parts of the world outside the United States. At one staff celebration, our staff represented Russia, Indonesia, India, Mexico, Cambodia, Africa, New Zealand, and America. The celebration included a potluck dinner, and the food was absolutely amazing.

The diverse care staff members have brought their reverence and respect for the elderly from their heritage. They are loving, caring, and hardworking, and they show a natural respect and admiration for the elderly population. This cultural perspective is a great asset for this industry.

Hiring the Right Person for Private Elderly Care

Many families initially hire care staff for Mom or Dad in the home before exploring alternative care options, such as assisted living, and they find themselves encountering the difficult task of hiring the right person. After investigating the essentials, such as a personal background check and previous similar work experience, further questions to consider before hiring someone include:

1. Will this candidate fit with the personality types of family members?
2. Will this candidate work hard and be ethical?
3. Will this candidate show up for work and not randomly call in sick?
4. Can this candidate manage his or her time to do the tasks required?

Missy Finds Purpose

Missy, our marketing director, was previously employed at a fancy hotel in town. She had been successful as a sales representative for the hotel, and her glamorous job had included coordinating events for executives. However, her job was "just a job," and she felt that she lacked a purpose or mission at work.

Missy noticed that her sister loved her nursing job, helping and caring for people. She would boast to Missy how her job was filled with a purpose that she enjoyed. Missy admired the health-care profession and individuals in these positions that combined a job with a meaningful purpose. In her free time, she became a volunteer for the elderly, and she found her volunteer activity more fulfilling than her hotel marketing job.

Eventually, Missy took a big risk and quit her high-paying job in sales to enter the assisted living industry as a marketing director. She took a pay cut because of the job change, and in the assisted living industry, she worked longer, harder hours with more pressure. However, the tradeoff was worthwhile for Missy. She enjoyed the endless learning experiences in her new work at a health-care community. She helped other people find a care environment for their mom or dad, and this position offered a great fulfillment of purpose for her.

During Missy's first days at her new job, she was afraid of the residents who had high levels of memory loss, and she did not know how to interact with them. Her previous volunteering activities did not prepare her for the extreme care situations of these residents. However, she received on-the-job education and training in elderly care and became familiar with the residents. As a result, Missy became comfortable discussing health care with the elderly population and their families. She learned what they needed for care and whether or not our community was the proper fit for them.

With Missy's new work and meaningful purpose, she could not wait to come to work. The elderly residents loved her, and they became like family to her. Missy occasionally put her marketing responsibilities aside to chat and help in the care of the elderly residents. When she was not at her desk, I occasionally had to search the community for her and found her with other care staff doing nails, makeup, and massages for the residents.

There are many people like Missy in the world outside assisted living who are waiting for an opportunity to add purpose to their lives. When we advertised for the Assistant Living Director position, we were overwhelmed by many Master of Business Administration (MBA) applicants who had been working in other jobs but wanted to enter a purposeful profession. These candidates were willing accept a salary cut of more than 50 percent to change to a more meaningful, fulfilling career.

Trusting the Assisted Living Community

When searching for the best assisted living community, it is important to have trust and confidence in the staff to care for a beloved parent. This trust develops from:

» discussions with other families and residents in the care community;

» the adult children's vision and expectations for good care;

» observations of the caring of those present in the community on tours or visits;

» consistency between claims about quality of care and results, assessed by state surveys.

It is important to learn as much as possible about the care community before making a decision. A gut feeling may give signals about an assisted living community and may help in the search for a good match for Mom or Dad.

It is also important to carefully evaluate the efforts of the team in the care of Mom or Dad. As a community administrator, I look for team leaders with enthusiasm and commitment, who enjoy working with elders. They should have integrity, and I must trust them to do the right thing in any circumstance. I surround myself with competent people who know how to collaborate in positive, creative ways. If they do not understand something, they must be comfortable asking questions, learning, and reliably following through. Many people are unaware of their own potential or do not know how to reach their desired goal. I like to use a positive approach of leading by example. With hard work and perseverance, people rise to the occasion with the right guidance.

Teaching by Example

Residents in the assisted living community may be accustomed to fine dining, cleanliness, and comfortable standards of life. The care staff members from diverse cultural backgrounds are required to provide services that may differ from their own experiences.

Teaching the diverse care staff by example is the key to success in combining cultures.

My personal approach to the assisted living community has been to come to work early, don an apron, and join the care managers in taking orders and serving breakfast in the dining room. I am familiar with fine-dining routines, food presentation, menus, taking orders, and serving. Most care staff members from different countries take great pride in home cooking and entertaining; however, the restaurant experience is not a cultural standard for many staff members, and they are not familiar with the details of this experience. Therefore, I created a protocol designed for care staff members who were not familiar with restaurant-style serving. Staff members work the dining room by my side to learn from my example.

The Best Steak

In a perfect world, all alternative care communities would provide great care. Although we do not live in a perfect world, adult children should expect excellent care for Mom or Dad. The care community may not be perfect, but it can deliver a standard of excellence that is achieved with constant reevaluation and adjustment of procedures.

Each restaurant has its own recipes and standards to provide the best menu, but the customer provides input with comments and feedback or by not returning for another meal. The alternative care community needs similar feedback about the care provided for Mom or Dad, and modifications may be made to improve the quality of care delivered. Feedback about poor care may be given to the caregiver immediately so that prompt adjustments can be made. In extreme situations, when the care is poor and not improved despite feedback, the resident's family may decide to move elsewhere.

If steak was important to a person, where would he go to

get the best steak? How far would he drive? How much would he spend? Restaurants that are known for the best steak will get the customer's business even if they are expensive. It is similar for people who search for the highest quality of care.

In deciding about the best place for Mom or Dad to reside and receive care, considerations include the quality of activities provided, cleanliness, health services, food, and overall care. The appearance of the care community is important but not the deciding factor. Adult children may travel far to find the best care environment for their parents. Price and available funds are always deciding factors for families because funds may diminish with time.

The Value of First Impressions

The alternative care community has only one opportunity to make a first impression. It is important for families to make note of initial observations during the first tour and ask the following questions:

» How are the residents dressed? How is their general appearance?

» What is the community's reputation?

» What are the results of family and state surveys?

» What do members of other families say about the community?

» What is your gut feeling about the environment of the community?

After several months with Mom living at the alternative care environment, the adult children may conclude that this is not the best place for her. If this occurs, it is best to resume the search for another community. If Mom remains in a suboptimal community, the adult children will worry about her eating, bathing, or safety, and the stress of this worry may affect their health and well-being. The next search may be more successful because the adult children will have more experience, wisdom, and awareness when selecting a new care environment.

When the Patient Is Right

Alice and her mother, Sue, visited our assisted living community. Sue entered with her walker, taking slow steps, and she appeared short of breath. When I asked how I could help them, Sue explained that she wanted to move from her current assisted living community. She complained that she could not get enough help from the staff because they were always busy.

Sue also shared that she wished that somebody could fix her voice. She spoke with a soft, raspy voice and cleared her throat many times. I explained that her voice may or may not be the problem, but there also might be a health condition that was causing her to feel short of breath and speak differently. With her permission, I checked her blood pressure and pulse, and I listened to her lung sounds. Although her blood pressure and heart rate were normal, I heard fluid in her lungs.

I was worried about Sue's condition and recommended that Alice take her to see a doctor. They called Sue's physician from my office and scheduled a doctor's appointment for the next day. I proceeded with the tour of our assisted living community, but I insisted that Sue use a wheelchair to minimize stress and exertion.

Sue returned to her previous assisted living community, and Sue and Alice showed the nurse-on-duty a note about the health-care issues and concerns that we discussed on her visit and tour. The nurse did not agree that Sue was ill, and she said that Sue did not need to see the doctor. However, Alice decided to keep Sue's appointment with the doctor because she wanted to be sure that Sue was healthy.

At the doctor's office the following day, it was determined that

Sue had pneumonia and may have had a stroke. She was admitted to the hospital straight from the doctor's office. Sue and Alice concluded from this experience that it was extremely important to have proper health care in the assisted living community, and that the health care in the previous care community was not sufficient. After discharge from the hospital, Sue moved to the new assisted living community.

Hole in the Wall

Years ago, I worked at a privately owned skilled care community ("nursing home") outside of Boston. This community was very basic in appearance, sterile as a hospital, and lacked a warm and inviting atmosphere. It was a "hole in the wall," needing much cosmetic improvement.

Despite its appearance, this care community was always full. Although it did not appear as pretty or modern as other nursing homes, it was renowned for having the best care in the area. We established ourselves as having the best of what people were seeking in a nursing home: an exceptional, high level of health care. We were full for no other reason.

Follow in My Footsteps

Later in my career, when I was working in another assisted living community, a consultant, Carol, shadowed me in my job. She wanted to experience the assisted living environment to help her learn to support other communities in developing policies and procedures. She had already visited other assisted living communities and had acquired most of the information that she needed. She had planned to shadow me for one to two hours because she wanted to see what we were doing in our community.

When Carol arrived at 10:00 a.m., I was busy with numerous issues and tasks of a typical Monday morning. In addition, the concierge had called in sick, and the telephones did not stop ringing. We had a new manager in orientation that needed training. Many residents were ill and needed arrangements for appointments and transportation to hospitals and doctors. Furthermore, it was the last day in November, and our staff members were decorating for the holidays with wreaths, lights, and Christmas trees. My busy day had started at 7:00 a.m., and I was already mentally fatigued when Carol arrived.

We began a simple tour, but Carol had endless detailed questions that required long explanations. With each new topic about the community, she added more questions. I struggled to juggle the time with her and the other operations, and her initially scheduled short visit occupied the entire day.

Carol became increasingly focused on our care and how it had evolved to such high quality in this care community. She was impressed that staff members repeatedly told her that they loved their job and would never want to leave. Carol witnessed a setting in which individuals were overqualified for their position, many having higher degrees or experience, but they had chosen this job because of the mission of giving. She saw a common thread throughout the community—that staff members felt loved and respected at work, and this made this community special and successful. She observed the loving care provided to the elderly residents.

Although my visit with Carol required much of my attention on a very busy day, her fresh view and comments taught me about the key components of the best assisted living environment. Although it is important for staff members to transfer a resident correctly and order the correct products, the most important element is the delivery of loving care. When Carol left at 5:00 p.m., she gave me a hug and thanked me, but I was grateful to her for giving me a better awareness of why our community had earned such a great reputation.

State Surveys

The state survey is an annual inspection by the state government to ensure that adult living communities are safe and properly organized. Every state has regulations about regular surveys of assisted living communities. During the state survey, one or two surveyors evaluate every aspect of operations and care in the community. It is the equivalent of taking a very difficult test for two days. Some communities view the state survey as a brutal but necessary experience. The surveyors:

» watch how care is given and check the ratio of staff members to residents;

» interview staff members, residents, and families to evaluate satisfaction;

» check medication records and physician orders to confirm correct implementation;

» evaluate meal preparation and food standards;

» inspect the environment for cleanliness and safety standards.

Although unpleasant and stressful, this regulatory scrutiny focuses the adult-care industry on quality assurance and promotes higher standards of quality and safety.

Request a Copy of the State Survey

When searching for an alternative care community for Mom, adult children should request a copy of the state surveys. After the annual survey is completed, the community receives a report that outlines issues of concern. "Deficiencies" are specific points that are not in compliance with state regulations and must be fixed. When a deficiency is cited, a plan of correction must be submitted within a designated time, and a follow-up visit is arranged to ensure that the plan was implemented successfully.

To recognize a good assisted living community from the state survey, the following observations can be considered:

1. Is the community administrator **proud to share the state survey** or does he or she avoid the subject?

2. Note the **seriousness of the deficiency issue** for which the community was cited. An excellent community may have deficiencies cited, but these deficiencies may be minor, for which the surveyors had to dig deep into details because there was no major or more serious deficiency present. Serious deficiencies affect the quality of health of residents, such as inadequate staffing, serious weight loss of residents, or a high frequency of falls. Minor deficiencies may include delays in completing educational standards or minor operational repairs.

3. Be **familiar with the issues that needed correction,** identified in the written state survey. During the tour, ask if these errors were corrected. Mom or Dad may be best served in an assisted living community that tackles problems properly and promptly.

The Wrong Fit

Despite a careful search for an alternative care community for Mom or Dad, the chosen community might be the wrong fit. An excellent community may be a wrong fit when the community cannot exceed customer expectations. When Mom or Dad has specific needs in daily care, the community may independently identify and provide the care needed.

The care community should keep the family informed about any changes in care, especially when care is increased or decreased. When a family member makes specific requests, he or she should confirm that the request was accomplished. However, in some instances, the proper care is not provided, and the community cannot get the job done. In these cases, the care community may not be the best fit, and the family may be directed to find a different setting that can provide the care required.

In one case, a son placed his parents in my assisted living community after receiving the advice from a referring nurse in another community. The initial demands of a quick admission seemed easy, and staff members worked after hours to prepare the apartment. However, the demands from this family were endless, and the expectations were not possible in the assisted living setting. The family demanded my personal availability, even when I was away or on vacation. The family had unrealistic expectations that were beyond the abilities of the community, such as full-time one-to-one care. Therefore, the family chose to take their parents elsewhere because our community was the wrong fit.

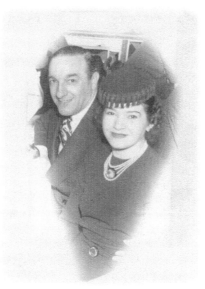

CHAPTER 11

Challenges Faced When the End Is Near

When Hospice Helps

Hospice care is an important part of health care for elderly people who are approaching the end of their life. It provides comfort to the person who is close to death and prepares the family for the loss of a beloved member. The usual focus of health care is to get well, so it is an adjustment for the assisted living resident and family to prepare for death.

When efforts are not working to help Mom or Dad feel better or get well, many people realize that hospice services are needed. Families may become exhausted from the 911 calls and trips to the emergency room for more pokes with needles. They recognize that the progressive degeneration cannot be cured.

Mom and Dad may prefer to decline peacefully, as written in their living wills. However, the family may not be ready to accept this wish. The alternative care staff may have the task of bringing the awareness of the need for hospice care to families. The staff may help the family recognize that Mom or Dad want to be kept comfortable and supported in the end-of-life experience.

The hospice mission of care is to coordinate a comfortable end-of-life experience for Mom or Dad and family. Hospice services have health-care staff members who curtail unnecessary tests and other measures that may interfere with a natural progression to the end of life. In the United States, Medicare pays for hospice services, but the patient must qualify with a terminal diagnosis or major decline, such as major weight loss, metastatic cancer, or heart failure.

Hospice services are initiated only on the order of a physician. The doctor discusses hospice care with Mom or Dad and the family. If Mom, Dad, or the person with power of attorney agrees, the physician refers Mom or Dad to the hospice health-care team. The hospice sends admission (intake) personnel to meet with Mom or Dad and the family, and they set care goals to guide all involved through the end-of-life experience.

Mom or Dad may remain at the alternative care community during hospice care. The hospice workers come to the community for care. If the person's needs cannot be met in the community, such as short-term symptom management issues, they are transferred to an inpatient hospice center and then returned to the community when the issue is resolved. Many comfort medications are immediately started by the hospice team, including medications to improve pain and sleep. The staff members in the alternative care setting work closely with the hospice team and allow the hospice to lead the end-of-life care. The alternative care staff members continue to provide hands-on care, and the hospice provides guidance, support, and counseling. Hospice staff members guide family and the alternative care staff in the comfort and other supportive measures that promote dying with dignity.

The alternative care staff members must adjust treatment goals to achieve comfort and not cure. The wellness approach from assisted living staff may be in conflict with a "comfort only" approach from the hospice staff, but both parties have the best of intentions.

In some situations, a health-care intervention, such as antibiotics, may seem the more comfortable route in managing a painful symptom, instead of pain medication alone. Open dialogue with family and health-care professionals may resolve differences of opinion and provide a unified approach for comfort measures used in the end-of-life care.

To Do or Not to Do

Assisted living nurses and hospice staff may differ in opinion about the most comfortable approach to pain management. Joan was a nonverbal resident with advanced dementia who was receiving hospice services. It was difficult to accurately assess and accommodate pain management because she was not able to speak. The staff members did not know her feelings or pain level. Her assisted living nurse and hospice staff member disagreed about the best pain management for her comfort level.

The situation became more complicated as additional health-care professionals, such as the hospice personnel, became involved and attempted to interpret her comfort needs. Hospice and assisted living staff subjectively attempted to analyze and interpret Joan's nonverbal messages, but each staff member had a different opinion about her pain source and intensity.

All staff and family agreed to make Joan's end-of-life experience as pain-free and comfortable as possible. Joan's long-term heart failure led to hospice care for her end-of-life experience. However, she developed a cough and fever, and a radiograph confirmed an upper respiratory infection. Additional comfort measures were discussed, and the options included antibiotics and pain medication or pain medication alone. Antibiotic therapy could relieve the pain and discomfort from infection and fever, but pain management alone could improve comfort without prolonging her painful life.

After the family considered the options, they decided to give acetaminophen and pain medication without the antibiotic, to provide a quicker path to death. With this open dialogue and decision making between the family, hospice staff, and assisted living nurse, all supported Joan in comfort management until her death.

At the End, the Tide Turns

As Dad approaches the end of his life, he may have control over how he declines until death. At a certain time, he may turn off his will to continue living, and he may choose to have his life end. After he has made this choice, he will show physical signs of decline, eat less, fight infections poorly, and decline in vital functions until his body shuts down and dies.

However, some healthy residents may have a strong will to live and may not be ready to die. The following true stories illustrate how Mom or Dad's different desires can sustain the will to live or extinguish the flame of life prematurely.

Larry's Watchful Eye

A loss of purpose can destroy the will to live. Larry had been a brilliant, driven man in his younger years. However, he had lost one of his children when the child was six years old, and he had never recovered from this loss. At age eighty-seven, Larry had severe dementia with delusions. A frequent delusion that excited him included visions that his deceased son was playing nearby in the assisted living community. The dementia led Larry to believe that his long-dead child was very much alive and present in our community and playing there at all times.

Larry kept very busy watching the young boy at play. In Larry's mind, the young boy played primarily in the downstairs area. Larry became upset when he had to go upstairs to his apartment, because nobody would be watching his young son. Staff members offered to watch his son, but Larry was aware that nobody else could see the boy. Therefore, Larry cleverly asked what his son was doing or wearing; when the staff member answered incorrectly, Larry refused to relinquish his responsibility of watching his child.

After many years in the assisted living community, Larry's funds were running low. His family moved him to a less costly community out of state, closer to them. Larry was distraught about moving and was aware that nobody else could watch his child.

Soon after the move, I called the family to check on Larry. They explained that Larry had declined quickly after the move and died. The change of environment was fatal for Larry because he could not live without the delusion of caring for his young son. This delusion had given him a purpose to stay alive. When he was separated from his imaginary son, he lost his will to live.

Jan's Love for Her Family

A loving family can fuel the assisted living resident's will to stay alive. Jan was once a beautiful young woman and a talented dancer. She was a fifteen-year-old high school student when she met Troy. They fell in love and married at a young age. Troy became an engineer, and they raised three children together. According to their children, Troy and Jan had a deep and genuine love for each other, and they were perfect soul mates. Throughout their lives, they never separated and rarely argued.

Troy developed advanced Parkinson's disease with dementia,

and he had difficulty walking and eating. He declined quickly during his stay at the assisted living community and died from complications of his illness. Jan was alone without him for the first time since their youth.

I worried that Jan's will to live would diminish and she would follow her husband in death, but I was wrong. Although Jan was distraught over Troy's death, she had her three children, who gave her strength and purpose to stay alive. Jan was a strong person, and she replaced the pain of loss with the purpose of joy with her children and grandchildren. It was not until several years later that Jan's heart finally failed with poor health and she died.

Betty at the Gates of Heaven

Strength can come from a vision or belief that sustains Mom longer in life or releases her, allowing her to die. Betty was an assisted living resident who had a vision that gave her strength to stay alive longer. Her health had been rapidly declining because of liver failure. Although she was very alert, every major body system was failing, and she was placed on hospice services. She was weak, bedridden, and close to death.

Betty's only child, Jenny, was close to her mother and visited frequently. One Friday, Jenny visited and found Betty wide-awake but distraught. Betty explained that she had visited the gates of heaven just before Jenny arrived, and she had waited in line with other people. However, when it was her turn in line, she was turned away and told that she must return on Monday. When Jenny left her mother's bedside, she shared this story with staff members, and she did not know how to interpret her mother's vision.

Early the following Monday morning, I came to work and went straight to Betty's apartment. She was lying in her bed, breathing comfortably, but she died within an hour. Evidently, her will to live had been influenced by her vision. She was guided by the belief that she would go through the gates of heaven on Monday.

Losing Her Ability to Love

Judy's strength to live was fueled by her ability to love and provide support for others. She was a very happy, religious, and social person. Family and friends described her as innately good-hearted, giving, and happy. She loved people and God. Her entire life was devoted to the care of her six children, church, charities, and helping the world in a positive way. She greeted people with a smile, calling them "honey" or "dear," and felt a genuine love for anyone crossing her path. She had a twinkle in her eye and a spark to live.

While she stayed in the assisted living community, Judy developed memory loss and became less able to care for herself. After several years in the assisted living community, her family moved her to a less expensive care option. I worried that the stress of the move or loss of familiar caregivers would catalyze her decline and death, which I had seen with other residents. However, Judy did very well in the new setting and remained alive for another six to seven months before her decline. Her family and I discussed her situation and agreed that Judy's widespread love for others enabled her to quickly love and adapt to the new staff.

When I attended Judy's funeral service, I gained a deeper understanding of how Judy's genuine love for others helped her accept her situation so readily, but how it also led to her losing her spark for life. The service was packed with people who could not wait to connect with others and share stories about her. I sat next to a woman who had known Judy for many years and who reminisced about Judy's life and path with family and God.

This woman told me that Judy and her husband once had exorbitant wealth and happiness. However, in a series of unfortunate events, all their wealth was lost. The only wealth that remained was nonmaterial—the wealth of caring, loving, and giving—but that sustained them. They became missionaries and freely traveled the world by boat to help others. They raised their six children on the boat during these many years and showed these children the path of helping others with the gift of charity and love. When I heard this woman's reflections, I was overwhelmed by Judy's impact on so many people.

Judy's dementia eventually interfered with her capacity to feel true love for others, and this contributed to her decline in health. Judy's decline from dementia caused her to lose the strength she needed to fulfill a lifelong purpose of loving.

Carol's Attachment

A simple change of location may cause a loss of the will to live. Carol had resided for three years in our assisted living community. She was alert, but she required much physical care. Her family relocated to a town two hours away. Initially, the family drove to visit her because they did not want to move her. However, it was difficult for the family to continue the long drive because of traffic and time, and they decided to move Carol to a care community closer to their new home.

Several months after the move, the family called to tell me that the stress of the move had a catastrophic effect on Carol. Soon after the transfer, her health declined, and she died. I had hoped that Carol would have enough cognitive awareness and strength to manage the move and adapt to the new care staff and community, but this did not happen. The family was devastated, because the purpose for Carol's move was to facilitate frequent family visits. Instead, it caused an earlier death. They had underestimated Carol's connection to her assisted living community before her move, and the loss was too great for her to endure.

Brian's Choice

Brian was another resident who lost his will to live after moving to a new place. He was in his nineties, and he had a strong will and an intense personality. His mood and temperament became more volatile and reactive with age, making his care difficult.

Throughout his adult life before his decline with dementia, he had a strong presence and loud bellowing voice, and he was the life of every party. He was a big talker and womanizer, and he loved to travel to his beach property two hours away.

After he developed dementia and moved into the assisted living community, he became more abrasive and untamable by family and staff. He was vocal, short-tempered, and aggressive, swinging his arms at the staff, with profanities pouring from his lips. He was resistant to care many times and continued to rule the day.

The staff members addressed his challenging personality with redirection, listening, and endless patience. The family and staff knew that if he failed to adapt to our assisted living community, other communities of care would likely sedate him. However, sedation was the family's last resort for his safe care. They feared that sedation would cause him to lose the spark of life that kept him going.

As years passed, Brian's physical decline gradually robbed him of his joy of life. He became deaf and had to lip-read because hearing aids did not help. His legs became weak, and he became wheelchair bound. When he developed heart failure, he was placed in hospice for care.

One day, he complained of severe pain that went from his chest down to his stomach. The hospice staff and I agreed with the family to move him to the hospice center where he could be watched and managed closely until he was stable and without pain. Although the hospice staff and his family felt that Brian would return from the hospice center in a few days, I could tell by his eyes that he was giving up. He seemed aware of his fragile health and weak heart, and he seemed tired of fighting.

I watched as he was put on the gurney for his transfer to the hospice center, knowing somehow that it was the last time I would see him. Several days later, I received a call from Brian's family. After he left the assisted living community, he did not eat or get out of bed, and he gave up, having lost his inner drive to live. He died within four days of leaving our community.

Erma's Patience

Some assisted living residents prolong their death and remain alive, aware that their loved ones are not ready to see them go. Erma and David were married for seventy years. Erma was declining physically, and David was with her at every stage. He was in love with her and unable to let her go.

Erma knew David's grief and seemed to be holding onto life just for him. She was bedridden for weeks, and she was unable to eat well or sit up independently. She might have been more comfortable with hospice care, but David was not ready to discuss it.

As their nurse, I spoke to David several times about hospice care, and he eventually agreed to let her go. Erma had been living with David in a one-bedroom, assisted living apartment, but she did not recognize him any longer. David felt that Erma had become a physical remnant of the wife he once knew.

David wanted to know about hospice care from my perspective. I told him that the soul eventually leaves the physical body; although Erma's physical body was present, her soul was gone. He listened to me with a bowed head, and he seemed to want permission to think about what I had said to him.

David completed the emotional process of letting go and was ready for Erma's death. Perhaps Erma knew that David was finally ready for her to go, because she died the next day.

Ducks in a Row

Some assisted living residents have important matters to arrange, and this may provide strength to delay death. Ron wanted to make sure that care would be provided for his wife, Ilene.

Ron was very healthy when he moved to the assisted living community with Ilene, who was declining with dementia. He had cared for her at home, but he had been diagnosed with an aggressive cancer. He knew that he would need a place to care for Ilene after his death, and he chose our assisted living community. He continued to care for Ilene for several years at the assisted living community.

Eventually, Ron's health quickly declined. When he became aware that he would not live more than two months, he made every effort to have Ilene join the other residents at activities and meals. He also let the staff members take over Ilene's care so she would be accustomed to them after his death. Ron felt peace with others caring for Ilene, and she became comfortable socially with others. He died without worry about Ilene's care.

When Care Staff Feel the Loss

Family and assisted living staff members experience the difficult challenge of accepting and delivering end-of-life care. Sometimes the family accepts this reality more readily than staff members.

Families may accept the change to end-of-life care because they may have prepared themselves mentally when Mom entered the alternative care setting. Families may feel that entry to the alternative care environment outside the home marks the beginning of Mom's path of decline and, ultimately, the end of her life. In contrast, the staff members who provide care are trained and educated in a wellness approach, and they may find it difficult to change focus and provide only basic comfort measures.

Turning Off the Switch

I had been involved with Ellen's care for the five years that she lived in the assisted living community. She was extremely demanding with endless details of care, but I was able to successfully guide the staff to accomplish her every request. Ellen and I shared humor together, and she had the most amazing smile. When Ellen smiled, it was as if a light was turned on. Her laugh was penetrating, involved her entire being, and radiated to everybody in the room. When she was happy, everyone felt her happiness; when she was displeased, we all felt the intensity of her displeasure.

When she was eighty-seven years old, Ellen's entire physical condition was fragile. She had heart failure, arthritic joints, and lung problems that required several inhalers. Despite her poor physical health, her spark for life was so strong that it was electrifying.

Ellen had given me a small stone engraved with the word "forever." I placed this stone among the others in my office fountain, and the fountain water continuously trickled over it, reminding me of her. Ellen was pleased that her stone occupied such an important place in the fountain, and she made sure that it was there on every visit to my office.

One day, Ellen acquired an infection and required hospitalization. Her body was quickly overcome by the illness, and many of her body systems failed. She struggled to get back to good health because she wanted to return to our assisted living community, which she lovingly referred to as her home. However, after the hospital stay, she was required to spend a short time in a skilled nursing home for more therapy.

In the nursing home, the domino effect of failing body systems led to further heart failure, and she was rushed back to the hospital. In the emergency room, she suddenly decided that she was ready to die, like turning off a switch. Ellen shared these feelings with her family, and they called me to tell me of her decision. However, my staff and I were not ready for her death. I recall glancing at the "forever" stone that she had given to me and realized that it signified her eternal drive to live.

Ellen was admitted to the hospital for end-of-life care. Hospice services were ordered, and all medications were stopped at her request. I visited her in the hospital and saw that she was struggling for each breath. Ellen had always been immaculately kept, with hair, makeup, jewelry, and outfits that were coordinated and fit just right; however, in her hospital bed, she was wearing a hospital gown, she had no jewelry or makeup, and her uncombed hair was pushed upward off her face. I attempted to see the person beyond the physical changes, but the spirit that once lit up the room was now dim.

As I struggled to accept Ellen's new end-of-life course, I noticed that many family members present were composed and accepting. Family members were discussing the day's events without emotion. I held back tears and avoided talking, for fear that my emotions would overtake me, and I would be the only person in the room crying.

I was not able to accept the fact that Ellen was ready to die, even though the family had accepted it. They understood, when she first entered the assisted living community, that her life was declining and that she would eventually die. However, the staff members and I kept Ellen in good health for five years in the assisted living community, and it was difficult to turn the switch off and begin the process of letting her go.

I was sad that Ellen had no will to live, because I had the will for her to live. I had one final conversation with her and whispered in her ear that I hoped that she was comfortable. She opened her eyes and gazed lovingly at me, which I took to mean, "Yes." I told her that we were here for her and we loved her, and I said my good-bye.

Within a few hours, I received the call that Ellen had died. She was at peace, picked her time, and moved on. She left me with great memories and a stone in my fountain that says "forever."

CHAPTER 12

The Reality of the Golden Years

The period of life after retirement has been referred to as the "golden years." Many elderly people find that their aging bodies fail, and this period may be overrated and not so "golden." Many aged adults, entering their eighties and nineties, struggle with physical decline, and they support their ailing health and mobility with medications and assistive devices, such as walkers and wheelchairs. People in this age group are the main supporters of health-care providers, including medical doctors, chiropractors, and acupuncturists.

Some people reflect on a world changing with time, contending that retirement is not what they had envisioned. They may have wanted to tour the country in a recreational vehicle, but they have developed difficulties driving. They had planned to travel around the world, but they cannot fly long distances because they have developed blood clots. They wanted to spend time with the grandchildren, but the grandchildren have moved to different countries. People are living, on average, five or ten years longer than in the past. Some people are in better health than similarly aged people in past times. Nevertheless, the health of elderly individuals in their eighties and nineties may worsen.

Years ago, grandparents frequently were in their late sixties or seventies, retired from their jobs and living a simple life. Many were mentally intact and very connected to the family, living close to their children and grandchildren. Now grandparents may live into the eighties and nineties, and they have an active life of their own with other seniors in addition to their family. However, poor health may limit activities with family or other seniors.

Many elderly people are struggling with the challenges of their physically aging body. Some who find true value in old age are at peace with their life challenges and enjoy the lessons of experience. For many people, the evolution of life may progress physically, emotionally, and mentally as follows:

» In the late teens to the early twenties, many people focus on improving physical appearance to be attractive and socially appealing. They begin building accomplishments for their résumé of life and focus on developing careers, excelling academically, and participating in sports and clubs. Many are driven to improve themselves and may be less focused on helping others. Many people are curious, careless, and carefree, with a young, resilient body.

» In the midtwenties to forties, many people acquire bigger possessions, such as a car or house, often with a partner or family. Life is focused on acquiring and achieving more and pursuing a family, job or business, social status, money, and possessions.

» In the late forties through sixties, many people have a midlife crisis, and they reevaluate their current situation and plans for the future. They may reflect and search for explanations to justify the purpose of their hard work.

Many people ask whether they want more, have too much, or are obtaining satisfaction with work and life experiences. Some people question whether they have acquired too many material things, as if they had eaten too much at a meal. Material objects may no longer satisfy their needs, and they search for purpose and meaning. However, others continue to consume and spend, leaving little in savings for future care. The body may show signs of aging and degenerative changes, including gray hair, wrinkles, and health problems. Many do not have the physical endurance that they had in the past. However, others may begin a wellness program, including attention to diet, supplements, and exercise, and they may improve their endurance and activities.

As people approach retirement, many search for new pursuits and hobbies to replace work. Individuals are happiest in retirement when they embrace life's rewards over the challenges. In the seventies, many people notice some physical decline and need increased physical maintenance. The mind may be intact and sharp, and many are at peace with the world and themselves. These early years of older age may be a period of reflection, a culmination of a life journey, during which material objects may become less relevant and the simplest elements of a day in one's life may be most meaningful.

In the late years of aging, most aspects of life require maintenance, and many people frequently need others to help with daily care. During this period, some people ask the question, "What is so 'golden' about the 'golden years'?" These years may be less about the physical enjoyment of life and more about viewing the world in a positive perspective and embracing life's accomplishments. The collection of life's memories and experiences creates wisdom. Many elderly people can appreciate and relish these memories. Others may spend their days complaining about poor health, loneliness, or poverty, or they may lose their memory and independence.

Rosie's Enjoyment

Rosie was 102 years old and in fair mental condition. She and her husband had raised three girls. She had fourteen grandchildren and great-grandchildren. She was admired by many people because of her longevity and health. She had witnessed many changes, having lived through the evolution of cars, telephones, and computers. She had acquired possessions that many people desire, including multiple homes, vacations homes, and nice cars. Yet her enjoyment of life in old age was not related to the possessions she had acquired.

Rosie was fortunate to experience old age with memories and cumulative love from a lifetime of family relationships. She explained that her family was most important to her, not the clothing business that she and her husband had successfully developed. She lived each moment for the connection with her children, grandchildren, and great-grandchildren. Although she was wheelchair bound and needed assistance for most physical activities, her memories remained fresh. She was clear that her family made her life so special. Her happiness and peace came from the simple enjoyment of those who loved her and those whom she loved.

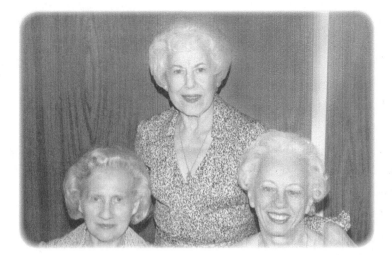

CHAPTER 13

Dodging Dementia

Family members or caregivers may worry about themselves declining and developing dementia. They have witnessed the decline of people with dementia, and they want to avoid this path themselves. They do not want to be dependent on others in their final years because of mental deterioration.

I overheard several members of the care staff discussing this worry. They asked one another about who would care for them if one of them began to lose their memory. They embraced one another in friendship and respected one another's experience in caring for people with dementia. They made a commitment to care for one another if they themselves developed Alzheimer's disease or other types of dementia.

The care staff had organized this plan in advance, to sustain themselves and minimize the disruption to their families. In some cultures, the elderly choose to alleviate the burden to others by connecting with nature for an end-of-life experience. Prevention, if possible, is the best course of action to address potential physical and mental decline and dementia.

Keeping mentally intact and sharp can be accomplished by participating in lifestyles that keep our minds and bodies active and fit. Eastern civilizations are familiar with this concept and include healthy lifestyles in their culture. The philosophy of a holistic lifestyle includes improving mind, spirit, and physical well-being. This is accomplished with daily meditation, a healthy diet, and daily physical exercise. In the early mornings during a visit to China, I saw parks filled with people who were gathering for meditation and other exercises for mind and body, including Tai Chi. The Chinese tour guide was in his late eighties, and I was amazed at his flawless memory and physical health that challenged mine at half his age. This mental and physical harmony in health may prevent the decline of the mind and dementia.

Prevention of dementia includes:

» Daily physical exercise. A study from Rush University showed that total daily physical activity decreased the risk of developing dementia by approximately 50 percent (Buchman, A. S., et al. 2012. Total daily physical activity and the risk of AD and cognitive decline in older adults. *Neurology* 24; 78:1323–9).

» Maintaining a healthy body weight. A study from Korea showed that people who were overweight or obese had a 2.2-fold to 2.4-fold greater probability of developing dementia (Chang, W. S., et al. 2012. The relationship between obesity and the high probability of dementia based on the body mass index and waist circumference. *Korean Journal of Family Medicine* 33:17–24).

» Nutritional supplementation. A study from Johns Hopkins University showed that daily supplementation with vitamin E (400 IU) and vitamin C (500 mg) decreased the risk of developing Alzheimer's disease by 78 percent. Furthermore, other studies have shown that folate and omega-3 fats may decrease the risk of stroke, a cause of dementia (Zandi, P. P., et al. 2004. Reduced risk of Alzheimer disease in users of antioxidant vitamin supplements: the Cache County Study. Archives of *Neurology* 61:82–8).

» Coffee drinking in midlife may decrease the risk of developing dementia by 65 percent. (Eskelinen, M. H., et al. 2010. Caffeine as a protective factor in dementia and Alzheimer's disease. *Journal of Alzheimer's Disease* 20 [Supplement 1]:S167–74).

Other factors may be helpful in preventing dementia, including:

» stimulation of the mind,

» limiting exposures to chemicals and molds,

» eating a healthy diet,

» participating in purposeful mind activities.

People who have a purpose in life typically keep their "spark" for living stronger, and they have the will to be more driven and empowered. Others who lose purpose in their life may lose motivation and energy that is necessary to maintain physical health and mental well-being.

Keeping the Spark

The challenge for everyone is to find a meaningful purpose in life. We all have a purpose that is unique to us and keeps us driven, but this purpose can change. This purpose may be a combination of giving, participating, and feeling valued.

Many women who are now in their later stages of life found

their purpose in being the caretaker of their home and family. After the husbands died and the children moved away, they suddenly had no more purpose. They either developed a new purpose or became depressed and ill. Many men had their purpose in their work and supporting a family; when they retired, they either found a new purpose or became depressed and unmotivated.

After one parent dies, the other may die within several months. This is not a coincidence, because some long-term couples have their life purpose interconnected. Identifying the purpose that is meaningful to Mom and Dad will help them maintain their emotional and physical health.

Sharpening the Mind

Mental acuity can be maintained by challenging the mind. The brain should be exercised as if it were a muscle. After sitting for a long period of time, a person may go for a walk to help maintain muscle tone and flexibility. Similarly, the unused mind needs a stimulating mental challenge to help maintain mental functions. Mind-engaging pastimes, such as games, puzzles, or reading, challenge the mind and exercise the memory to help preserve brain function.

Stay-at-home moms occasionally seek playgroups for their child, both for the child's interaction and their own mental stimulation with other adults. Dad may obtain his mental stimulation from watching the History Channel, playing cards, or pursuing a hobby.

Some people work into their seventies or eighties, but their minds begin to fail after retirement. The mental stimulation from the work environment had not been replaced, and they neglected to have the brain engage in another type of mental exercise.

Some cases of apparent memory loss actually may be a result of emotional withdrawal from interacting with others because of boredom or depression. In these cases, Dad may become more alert, and his memory may improve, when he awakens the mind with mental stimulation.

A Trip to the Past

Kip was an assisted living resident who had moderate memory loss that affected his short-term memory primarily and his long-term memory slightly. When his daughter, Terra, was getting his home ready to sell and was cleaning out the basement, she stumbled on a stack of original newspapers from 1939 to 1950. She brought the newspapers to Kip, and he read the newspaper headlines and articles out loud for a group of residents. The group members were intensely interested because the articles ignited memories from the past, and people began to recall where they were at the time of the events in the articles. The newspaper session awakened long-term memories about these World War II events, and none of the residents seemed to have a memory deficiency. In fact, the residents were able to dispute the published commentaries about the events.

Physical Maintenance

The body is a vehicle that enables people to accomplish physical needs and desires, but poor physical health may limit the ability to accomplish these tasks. People who have limited use of the arms may not be able to eat well independently. Poor vision may limit the ability to read. People must keep their body healthy to maximize physical abilities.

To maintain optimal physical health, people require daily exercise, a healthy nutritional program, and attention to bodily needs. Listen to your body! If you are thirsty, drink water. If you are hungry, eat healthy food. If you are tired, get some sleep. Addressing the body's basic desires may help maintain physical health and strength.

Failure to pay attention to the body's needs may occur because of being overworked or eating for reasons other than hunger, and this may cause illness, fatigue, or stress. Eventually, the "wear and tear" may cause a person's physical health to decline, possibly resulting in high blood pressure, diabetes, cardiovascular disease, cancer, or obesity.

Some people put more effort into caring for their cars than their bodies. They change the oil, rotate the tires, and schedule tune-ups. A neglected car can be replaced, but a neglected body may suffer degeneration and chronic disease.

The Right Nutrients

A healthy nutritional program is vitally important to maintain physical health. This includes obtaining the right nutrients in optimal amounts and avoiding foods that can be harmful. Good carbohydrates that do not spike the blood sugar ("low glycemic") are obtained from most colored fruits and vegetables and some whole grains. Good fats include the omega-3 fats. Optimal amounts of nutrients cannot be obtained from a healthy diet alone, and the benefits of a high quality nutritional supplement program are supported by numerous published research studies. Frequent low-glycemic snacks help avoid hunger that may cause overeating at meals and sugar overload.

Many packaged foods are chemically modified and contain unhealthy additives and artificial ingredients. It is best to avoid artificial ingredients. Organic foods help minimize the exposure of the body to environmental toxins, such as pesticides that can cause disease.

Spiritual Health

The keys to building a strong inner self include a connection to personal values, feeling valued, and feeling loved. Inner self is the force inside a person that gets him or her out of bed in the morning and provides the strength to seize the day. It may seem easier to identify and address issues about physical health than to measure the health of the inner self.

A weak inner drive may cause a lack of motivation and may weaken the immune system, increasing susceptibility to infection. The inner strength is tested during a life crisis, such as a diagnosis of cancer, death in the family, or divorce. These times of crisis force an individual to tap into the inner strength. If the inner strength is weak, then the person will have difficulty coping. The inner self may be strengthened by maintaining loving and caring connections.

A strong sense of community may strengthen the inner self and provide support during a crisis. People can become stronger physically when they have motivation and determination from a strong sense of self. This community support can be developed through connections with religious groups, family, or friends. Meditation can increase self-awareness and strengthen the inner self. When people are out of touch with their religious or spiritual self, they may have less inner strength to address the daily challenges of society.

Epilogue

When All Is Said and Done

We can best take care of Mom and Dad by seeking practical solutions to maintain health and manage symptoms. This is accomplished by learning as much as possible about them. By paying attention to their needs, we become aware of the "dos" and "don'ts" for their care. We learn to obtain the proper help and use available resources, both within and outside the family.

Adult children should not neglect their own needs when they are taking care of Mom and Dad. The consequences of neglecting these needs may be another crisis, such as a personal health issue. Family and caregivers can become educated about the symptoms and situations as they evolve. Excellent care does not require perfection and may be provided with thoughtfulness and the best intentions.

The road to taking care of Mom and Dad can take many surprising turns. The family members caring for an elderly person must brace themselves for an adventure that has no clear map for success. The basic elements that keep families intact when in crisis include love, support, and effective communication.

It is important to seek guidance from available resources and to trust the health-care professionals to satisfy Mom or Dad's care needs. When faced with the challenge of caring for Mom or Dad, the focus should be on tackling the care situation in the most prepared way possible. Mom and Dad may not understand the efforts of the family, and they may be unable to show appreciation, but they will be safe and cared for in the best manner possible.

INDEX

Guilt 5, 21, 60, 67, 155–160, 178

H

Hospice 18, 150, 152, 160, 201–204, 206, 209, 210, 212

I

Incontinence 8, 116–118

L

Lewy Body Dementia 11
Long-term memory 14, 59, 80, 81, 96, 107, 108, 141, 223

M

Medications 23, 40, 47, 49, 51, 52, 66, 70, 80, 83, 93, 100, 104, 112, 118, 127, 128, 129, 130, 132–134, 136, 137, 139, 141, 146, 149, 152, 202, 212, 215
Memory loss xiv, xv, xix, 4, 8, 10, 19, 22, 23, 25, 26, 31–33, 35–37, 39, 40, 45–47, 49, 50, 51, 53, 56, 58, 59, 65, 82, 83, 88, 95, 96, 103, 107, 108, 119, 120, 123, 132, 136, 159, 161, 162, 177, 178, 182, 187, 190, 207, 222, 223
Mental health 16, 52, 121
Mild memory loss 4, 35, 36, 39, 40, 45, 107
Moderate memory loss 45, 46, 50, 83, 88, 107, 108, 223
Mold 50, 51, 221

N

Nutrition xix, 4, 10, 12, 23, 54, 109–112, 121, 128, 130, 131, 137, 221, 223, 224

P

Parkinson's disease 66, 151, 152, 205
Physical care 10, 54–56, 208
Physical health xix, 48, 113, 121, 129, 132, 212, 220–225
POLST 146–152

S

Safety 1, 5, 6, 10, 20, 36, 39, 53–55, 57, 58, 60, 61, 71, 88, 93, 101, 121–125, 131, 134, 162, 175, 181, 193, 197
Severe memory loss 36, 46, 47, 107
Sexual behaviors 79–83
Spiritual health 224
Stage of dementia 27, 32, 34–36, 43, 46, 47, 55, 76, 89, 94, 103, 107, 117, 118, 178
State survey 191, 193, 197, 198
Sundown syndrome 70, 71, 93, 94

T

Toileting 11, 116, 118
Total care 33, 46, 47

V

Vascular Dementia 12
Visual abilities 112
Vitamin B12 13, 49

W

Wander Guard 66, 78

Contact Kathy!

Do you have a comment, question, or concern about your parents? Have they been diagnosed with dementia? Are your parents living in an assisted living community?

Write to Kathy J. Stewart at kathyjstewart@cs.com.